Body School

For all who suffer the human condition...

DAVID KNOX

BODY
SCHOOL

Meyer & Meyer Sport

British Library Cataloguing in Publication Data

A catalogue record for this book is available from the British Library

Body School

Maidenhead: Meyer & Meyer Sport (UK) Ltd., 2015

ISBN: 978-1-78255-058-7

© 2015 by Meyer & Meyer Sport (UK) Ltd.

Aachen, Auckland, Beirut, Cairo, Cape Town, Dubai, Hägendorf, Hong Kong,

Indianapolis, Manila, New Delhi, Singapore, Sydney, Tehran, Vienna

Member of the World Sport Publishers' Association (WSPA)

Total production: Print Consult GmbH, Munich

ISBN 978-1-78255-058-7

E-Mail: info@m-m-sports.com

www.m-m-sports.com

TABLE OF CONTENTS

INTRODUCTION

This book is about you and your body—how it works and how it breaks and how to get the best from one and the least of the other. Laid out in common language and specific detail, it is a guidebook to freedom of movement and freedom from pain.

Through these pages you learn how to think for your muscles, how to take the information you gather and use it to better understand and improve your body and better heal its injuries. You learn how to take the lead in your own physical destiny.

Though we are all made very similarly, we are no two exactly alike. This book will help you find your way; it will lead you to your right questions. The answers will be found in your muscles, joints, nerves and presence of mind.

ABOUT THE AUTHOR

For 41 years, I have worked in the world of professional physical arts. In the course of innumerable injuries to every part of my body, I have consulted with and been treated by a broad array of doctors, physical therapists, acupuncturists, chiropractors and others, with varying degrees of success. I have studied postural and therapeutic protocols—Western and Eastern, methodologies—mainstream and arcane, and I have come to certain conclusions about what works and what doesn't when it comes to healing, maintaining and, if you wish, getting the most out of that one item whose lifetime warranty is truly guaranteed—the human body.

My professional life began as a dancer, studying in New York in 1976, where I trained with some of the best teachers in the world. In 1988, I began studying martial arts, directly from the creators of two schools and, later, from the senior disciple of a third, earning two black belts. In accord with studying these disciplines, I received a strong education in the applications of strength, flexibility, massage as therapy, injury management and recovery.

Aside from performing, over the years I have taught classes—in yoga, power yoga, martial arts, self-defense, kickboxing, flexibility, ballet, exercise form and technique—and, for six years, I was a lead instructor in an outdoor boot camp. I continue teaching today and working as a personal trainer.

The fly in my ointment (and it's a Big Fly) was discovered when I was 24. That's when I was first seriously afflicted, and subsequently diagnosed, with a vertical, hairline fracture in my lower spine— what one might call a congenital birth defect.

When it shifts, a severe electric shock renders my legs useless, and I collapse to the floor. As many as six very painful weeks pass before I can walk again. Not willing to submit to the restrictions of spinal surgery, I have spent decades determining effective rehabilitation and maintenance strategies that keep me on my feet.

As an instructor, I have followed the same train of thought that evolved from understanding my back problems and applied the same analysis and recovery techniques to all kinds of injuries on all kinds of body types, from teenagers to octogenarians, with continued success. However, the greatest success comes when individuals learn to help themselves.

Indispensable to my education, and a great good fortune in my life, is my brilliant father, Dr. Murray Heimberg, who has worked in medicine for more than 50 years and taught me so very much about the physiology that is us.

REFERENCE INDEX

Numbers below indicate exercises and stretches, accessed by page numbers listed on the page opposite. These tables apply to both the healthy and the injured.

Location	Injury	Page	Exercise	Flexibility
Neck	The Neck	248	14, 15, 19, 23, (25)	1, 2, 6
Shoulders	The Neck and Shoulders	261	14-23	1, 2, 3, 5, 6, 16 ,19
	The Shoulders	269		13, 14, 15
Chest	The Chest	294	14, 15, 16, 17, 22	1, 2, 3, 10, 13, 14, 16, 19
Abs	The Abs	295	(25), 6-13	2, 4, 10, 13, 14, 16
Middle Back	The Middle Back	286	7, 8, 11, 12, 13, 14, 15, 18, 19, 23	1, 2, 3, , 5-13, 15, 16
Lower Back	The Lower Back	298	6-13, 18	4-15, 16
Hips and Buttocks	The Hips and Buttocks	312	1-6, 9-13	2, 4-13, 15, 16
Thighs	The Thighs	321	1-6, 9-13	2, 4, 9, 10, 12, 14, 16, 18
Knees	The Knees	327	1-6, 9-13	2, 4-13, 15, 16
Calves	The Calves	329	1-6, 9, 10, 13	2, 4, 5, 7, 8, 9, 12, 17
Ankle	The Ankle	335	1, 2, 3, 4, 5, 6, 9, 10, 13	2, 4, 5, 7-10, 12-15, 17
Foot	The Foot	337	(same as Ankle)	(same as Ankle)
Toes	The Toes	339	3, 5, 6, 9, 10, 13	4, 5, 7-10, 12, 13
Upper Arm	The Upper Arm	340	14-23	1, 2, 3, 6, 10, 13, 16
Elbow	The Elbow	342	14-23	2, 3, 5, 6
Forearm	The Forearm	343	14-24	2, 3, 5, 6, 10, 13, 16
Wrist	The Wrist	344	14-24	3, 5, 10, 13, 16
Hand	The Hand	351	14-24	1, 2, 3, 5, 6, 10, 13
Fingers	The Fingers	353	(same as Hand)	(same as Hand)

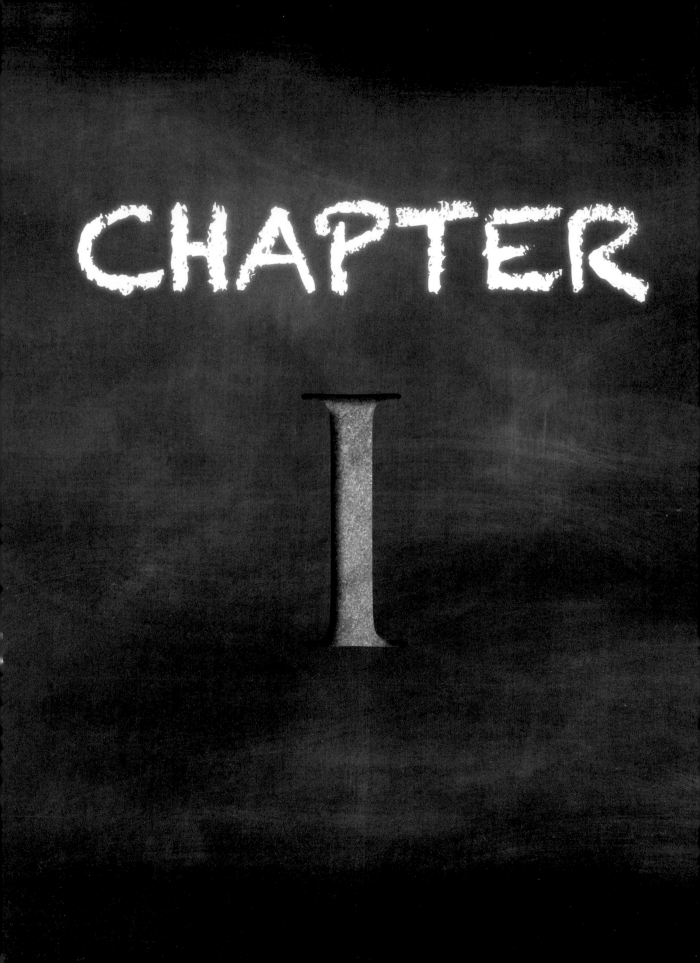

CHAPTER I: BEFORE WE BEGIN

In order to get from this book all that it has to offer, there are a few guidelines that must be followed.

THE FIVE LEARNING ESSENTIALS

1. First and foremost—Think! Although all of the guidelines listed here are equally important, without this first, the others have no chance. Thought, focus and intention are every bit as important in exercise as in any other aspect of life. It's your body—the only way to understand how it works is to make the work your own. So, think. Which brings us to our next rule:

2. Safety. Safety first, safety last, safety in the middle! It is my belief that there is a safe way to move the body in any way it has been built to move. Take your time, don't grow impatient and develop your technique properly. And that brings us to the next rule:

3. Precision. Know where your body parts are and put them exactly where you want them to be. You only have to be off just a little at the wrong time, or a little for a long time, to create an injury that won't seem to go away. Furthermore,

poor technique will deprive you of the full benefits of your work and reinforce negative habits. Remember, you're training your muscles. They can only learn to the degree that they are taught. Which brings us to our next rule:

4. Support. When you move or position your body, don't leave it up to your joints and bones to take the full load—use your muscles! Often, we only see the most obvious part of an exercise, not taking into account the support of the rest of the body. Once again, you decrease your benefits and increase your risk of injury without proper support. But don't take my word for it. Decide for yourself. Which brings us to our next rule:

5. Question. Question everything. Question everything that I say in this book, question everything that anyone, from the rankest amateur to the most acclaimed specialist, ever tells you about moving your body. If you don't understand the information, ask questions and think about it until you do. If you want to try something out, do so safely, with precision and support, and see how it feels. There are so many different ideas out there, so many different expert opinions, so much about the body that is still being discovered. It's up to you to find what works best for you.

A WORD ON MUSCLES

When you were a baby, you had to learn how to walk. As you toddled, you learned to guide food into your mouth. You learned to run, to reach, to throw, to jump—the list goes on and on. In every case, you first had to learn. The good news is, your muscles are waiting to be taught. They are genetically designed to learn the things you teach them to do. However, they rarely learn overnight, and the harder the task, the finer tuned the precision, the longer it takes.

So, patience is the key here—patience and dedication. Some things you try may be fairly easy, while others may prove considerably harder. Some things an instructor tells you that you should feel as you work, you may, at first, either not be able to feel at all, or be mistaken in what you think you are feeling. I still continue, to this day, with all my diligent training, to have occasional major physical revelations, in which I finally feel, for the first time, things I'd been taught years before, things I had thoroughly grasped, from the beginning, as concepts in my mind. My point is that just because your brain understands a physical instruction, that doesn't necessarily mean that you can make your body do it right off the bat. It takes practice, my friends. Anything's possible with thoughtful, dedicated practice. Don't like the way you walk? Shoulder not feeling right? Fix it with steady practice. Wish you were a better dancer? Practice.

Of course, we are all limited by our own personal genetics, and one person may excel where another shines but dimly. Yet, I don't believe that anyone is hopelessly uncoordinated. If you teach your muscles, they will learn. The biggest barrier to a person's learning is not one's physical inability, it's one's ego. Not wanting to try something you don't think you'll be instantly good at. No one likes to feel foolish, especially in front of others.

The thing is, don't worry about it. Relax. Everyone who has ever existed, when learning something new, has had to start at the beginning, from that poorly skilled, potentially embarrassing, even laughably bad place—the very place from which all good things may grow. The greatest athletes in the world had to start at that place, and, I assure you, many of them felt at least as silly as the least among us. Yet, they persevered, and, eventually, everything changed. So, when you try something new, try this also. Leave your ego at home. Concentrate on the work. No matter who you are, you will improve over time. Your muscles will learn.

A WORD ON JOINTS

Bones give our bodies a definitive form. Without bones, our bodies would be nothing better than quivering masses of muscles and organs lying blob-like on the floor, or taking the general shape of whatever vessel into which they might be poured. It's nice to have bones.

Joints in the bones allow our bodies to move. Cartilage, on the ends of and between the bones, cushions the joining. Reaching across the joints, attaching the bones to each other, are dense, fibrous ligaments. Overlapping the joints and ligaments, from either direction, are the muscles, supported and attached to the bones by somewhat tougher tendons. The overlapping muscles contract and extend to move the joints and keep them aligned and stable. Different joints do different things. The degree to which a joint can be safely moved in all the ways and directions for which it was designed is called its *range of motion (ROM)*.

Range of motion varies widely from one person to another and decreases with lack of use as muscles, tendons and ligaments lose their flexibility. It can also decrease as one ages, depending on the health of the joint and one's general level of fitness. The good news is, it can be redeveloped, or, at least, its deterioration considerably slowed, with a bit of safe and steady practice. Not all positions in a joint's range of motion are equal, however. Just because your body can move that way doesn't mean it should be heavily stressed in that position. Too much weight at the end of your range, too little support in the course of a movement, push a joint just a little too far (over-rotation/hyperextension) and zap!—it's too late. You're injured.

So, treat your joints kindly. Think about what they're built for; think about how they move. Think about how your particular joints line up; think about how they respond in different situations. When trying something new, observe carefully and gently control the entire operation until you're sure that your body understands. Never stress an unsupported joint or attempt to push it in a direction it was not built to go.

A WORD ON BODY TYPES

Bodies come in different sizes and shapes, each of which may have different pros and cons. Tall people may have more back problems, short people a more confined range of motion. The thicker among us may have a hard time getting thin, whereas some on the skinny may find it hard to gain weight. It has to do with how you were built and what you've built from what you were given.

Regardless of our individual models, the human body is built for action. We are descended from hunter-gatherers, people who chased the wooly mammoths across Iberia, or foraged barefoot in the jungles, or developed crops, by hand, in the Fertile Crescent. Advances in social technology aside, we are still built this way. To ignore this fact comes at a high price. Diminished physical abilities, diminished pleasure, chronic pain, weight issues, breathing problems, heart and circulatory risks—these are but a few—can all be brought on or made worse by not properly maintaining your body.

What you do with it is, ultimately, your concern. But, whether you work it because you want to, or only when you must to recover from or prevent a worse situation, anyone—tall, short, fat, thin, loose, tight, weak, strong—can achieve results. You may have to start very slowly and the road may seem impossibly long, but you can achieve results. Don't worry about the length of the road—just take it day by day, one step at a time. Be patient. You will amaze yourself.

Understand your body. Understand your strengths and weaknesses. If you can, find a health-building physical activity that inspires you and get to work. Just remember, as I often do, the words of Sensei Robert Bryner, master of Okinawan kempo and aikido, "Work on the hard stuff. The easy stuff is easy."

A WORD ON DIET

Do I really need to say it? You are what you eat. Food is either nutritionally rich or nutritionally poor, and your muscles (including your brain, my friends), bones, organs and everything else grow stronger or weaker depending on what you feed them. In automotive terms, the fuel and lubricants you put into your machine determines, along with maintenance, how well your machine works. Eating a diet rich in whole grains, fruits and real vegetables, lean proteins from meat, poultry, fish, dairy, soy, chickpeas, lentils, using unsaturated oils when you cook with oil, having some nuts along the way—this sort of thing will build your body, your mind and influence, in a big way, who you are. You'd be surprised how much diet can affect one's personality.

If losing weight is your intention, let me redirect your thought a bit. Losing weight should be a goal for many people who are obese, but obesity is defined as a percentage of body fat—over 25% for men and over 30% for women—not weight. So, when you say you want to lose weight, is that really what you mean? Two people of the same height and weight can vary drastically in their respective percentages of body fat. One could be lean and mean, bulging with muscle, the other saturated and fat, puddling with gravy. Providing the lean person is not using illegal steroids to gain size, would you say they both needed to lose weight? What about thin people with high body-fat percentages? They need something, but it's not losing weight—they just need to convert unhealtful fat to healthy muscle.

Muscle takes up, on average, one-third as much space as fat and creates a more dynamic image—strong and lifted versus heavy and earthbound, lean and shapely versus drooped and bony. I have seen many a svelte silhouette, many a strong posture and taller presence created when not an ounce of weight was shed. One woman I worked with, five days a week, one hour per day, lost seven inches off of her waist in six weeks though her weight did not change. The point is, many people who think they need to lose weight actually need nothing more than to burn their fat into muscle.

Still, if you're a lean size 7 and you want to make size 5 (and it can often be done healthfully), or you do have extra pounds you truly wish or need to shed—it's really simple—burn more fuel than you consume. Burn more calories (fuel) than you eat—you will lose weight. Eat more than you burn—you will gain weight. Regardless of all the exciting new diets out there, gaining and losing weight always begins and ends with calories. It's that simple, and it's that absolute. No two ways about it. Of course, there are many more specific and important things to consider in one's diet than just eating healthful foods and being aware of one's caloric consumption, but it's a good place to start. The good news is, there are any number of professionals, books and other sources available for your further research. If you really want to get serious, look into them. Good nutrition builds good stuff. Poor nutrition inhibits the growth of every good thing you've got. It's your choice.

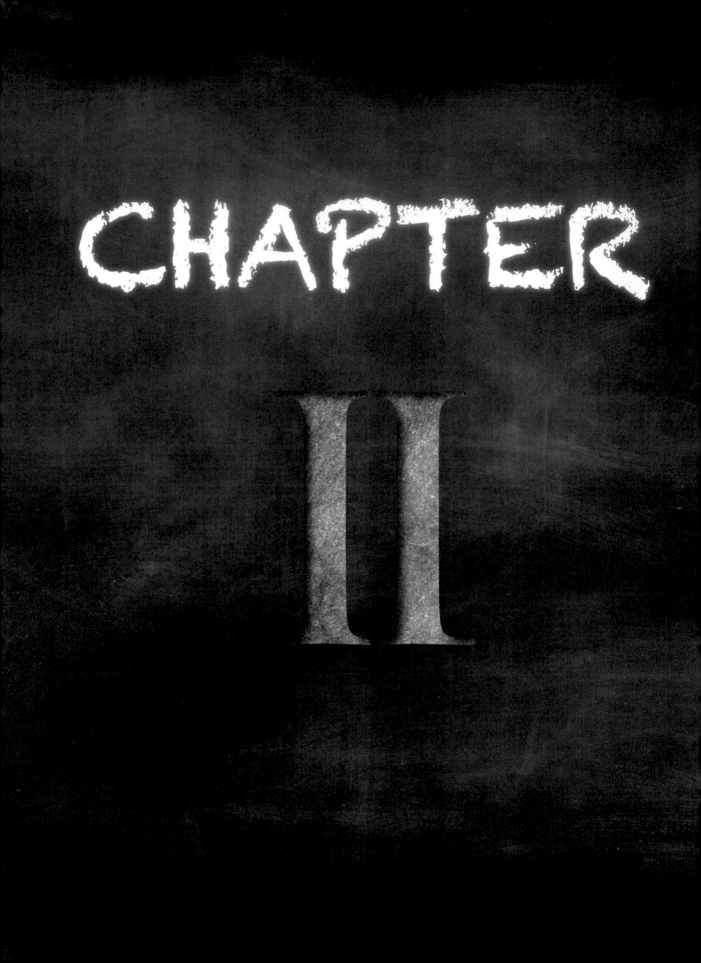

CHAPTER II:
FORM
(A GOOD PLACE
TO START)

In order to get a working sense of the individuality of your muscles and how they come together as a team, let's start off with something relatively simple, a little thing I like to call:

GETTING
TO KNOW YOU

Everything in your body is interconnected. Nothing happens without other things getting involved. Regarding your muscles and joints, nothing moves without several factors coming together. Various muscles must cooperate, the joints have got to be up for it, and the brain must send the right messages down the right nerves to the right receptors in the right muscles that have been trained to interpret the messages properly and produce the desired movement. Remember when you learned to write?

Even the movements of our everyday lives—walking, bending, sitting, reaching, grasping, going up and down stairs—are done in the ways we've trained our bodies, consciously or unconsciously, to do them.

Through these everyday movements, we've become relatively familiar with the larger muscle groups of the body. We feel the calves, thighs and butt when we squat, walk and climb; we feel the back and shoulders when we pull or lift; we feel the chest and shoulders when we push or press; and we feel the arms and hands when we push, grip, pull and lift.

Unfortunately, although we are all aware of the belly—which should be working in all of the moves mentioned previously—whether it actually gets involved or not varies greatly from one person to the next.

Still, none of our big guns would be very effective without the stabilizing and guiding assistance of smaller and lesser-known muscle groups.

TOES, FEET, ANKLES AND CALVES

Look at your feet. You stand on them, walk on them, press on them every day. Yet, when was the last time you thought about how they really work? Have you ever considered the various muscles in your feet and toes?

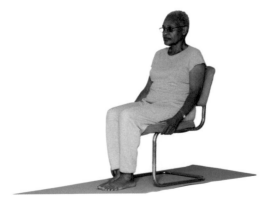

Sit down in an armless chair (not too cushy, one with support) and get barefoot. Then, sit up straight—don't arch—with your back solidly supported by the back of the chair. Arms relaxed by your sides; hands may gently grip the sides of the seat (Photo 1).

PHOTO 1

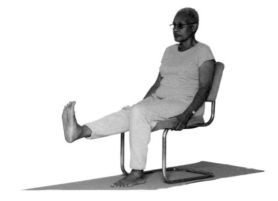

PHOTO 2

Stretch one leg out straight and flex your ankle (pull the top of the foot toward the chest). Now, try to pull your toes toward your chest (Photo 2).

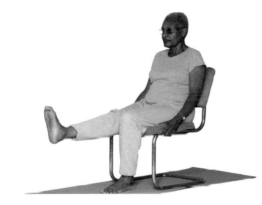

PHOTO 3

Feel anything extra? More squeeze in the front of the calf, maybe? More stretch in the back of the calf? Keep the foot flexed as strongly as you can and try to curl the toes down, as though you were making a fist (Photo 3).

Can you do it without moving the ankles? Feel the tops of the calves now?

Pull the toes back again and try to extend the feet, as though you were on tiptoes. Can you hold the toes back or do they reach forward with the ankles?

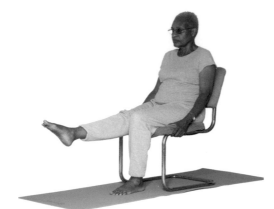

If you managed to hold them back, keep the feet extended and point the toes (Photo 4).

PHOTO 4

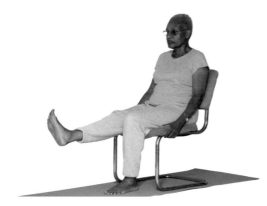

Do they really reach out or do they just curl down? Now, rotate them open and flex and point a couple of times (Photo 5).

PHOTO 5

You can train your feet to do any of these things and have stronger, more stable calves, feet and ankles for your effort. (If your feet cramp while pointing, pull the toes back or flex the entire foot. Work the feet regularly, and the cramping will eventually go away.)

Now grab a couple of marbles or similar small objects (bottle caps can work; coins are tougher) and drop them on the floor. Pick one up with your toes and extend your leg. While holding the object, point and flex your ankle. Think about the front of your calf and feel the muscles there when you flex. Really work your range of motion. Consider the top of the foot as it changes angles.

HIPS, KNEES AND THIGH ROTATORS

Release the marbles and lie down on your back on the floor, legs out straight and pressed together. Place your arms on the floor, diagonally from your body, palms down or, for an extra stretch, comfortably out over your head.

Stretch your legs out straight. Don't think, "Lock the muscles to hold the position", but rather think fluid strength, long and reaching, like your legs were two living, reaching steel beams (Photo 6).

Flex your feet and toes and pull those heels out long, away from the hips (Photo 7). Point and flex (full range) a few times.

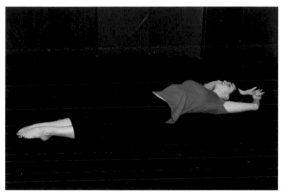

PHOTO 6

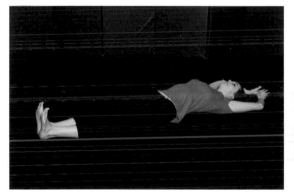

PHOTO 7

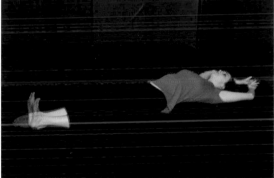

Now, squeeze your butt hard, keep your heels together and turn your knees open (Photo 8). The feet will naturally follow. The rotation occurs from the hips.

Stretch your legs, if you can, until the backs of your calves touch each other.

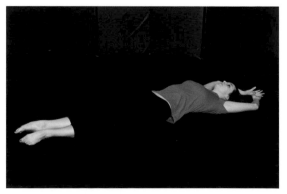

PHOTO 8

People with hyperextended joints must be careful, and everyone should be aware of any potential cramp in the muscles or pain deep inside or at the back of the knee.

As you use your butt to turn the knees out, do you feel the difference in your backside? Welcome to your rotators!

We've all heard of the *gluteus maximus*, but do you know the other members of the gluteus family? They come in three sizes—maxi, midi, and mini (and, coincidentally, ladies, do provide some padding for the body). Big Max, along with several muscles that lie underneath deeper in the backside, is largely responsible for rotating your legs in and out. It is from the hips that leg rotation is safely performed. Pity of it is, most people think from the feet up, rather than from the hips down, and their feet and knees go where they will. Not a good idea.

With your legs in open rotation, slowly flex and point the feet a few times, making full use of the toes. Do you feel the extra work in the butt and back of the legs when you flex the feet?

Think about the outside of the thighs, from the butt through the knee. Feel the outside of the calves as you move from point to flex. Mimic holding a marble with the toes as you flex.

Move the heels a few inches apart, keep your legs strong and try to rotate the feet around the ankles in a full circle. Try to use the toes as well, flexing them when the foot is flexed, pointing them when the ankle points. Work both directions, at least eight repetitions. Work regularly, and you will improve.

(You may have noticed, as you rotated your legs out and open, a stretched and tightening feeling at the sides of and beneath your lower belly. Along with the rotators in your butt, there are other muscles attached to the lower spine that reach down through your hips and help turn the legs. Being aware of them and using them consciously can really help trim a waistline and flatten a pooch.)

WORKING SUPINE STRETCH

Relax for a moment. When you're ready, interlace your fingers and stretch your arms out above your chest. Press your shoulders down into your body and down into the floor, squeeze your butt, rotate your knees out, stretch your legs, and either flex or point your feet and toes. Pull your chin in until you feel a stretch in the back of your neck and contract your belly down toward your spine.

Inhale slowly and deeply into the chest, as you reach with stretched arms, slowly, out past the top of your head and toward the floor, as far as is comfortable. From the hips down, you're reaching one way, from the shoulders up another (from the shoulders, not with the shoulders—don't let them get up around your ears—keep them in place!).

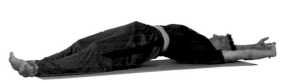

Try squeezing your butt up off the floor as you stretch (Photo 9).

PHOTO 9

And flatten that belly at the top!

Between the two stretches, the torso is working (keep that belly strong to protect your spine!). It's like pulling taffy.

As you exhale, refine the move and consider the details.

BRIDGE/PELVIC CURL

Moving on, let's go to an exercise commonly known as the bridge. It is taught lying on the back, with the knees bent vertically and the feet close to the hips, arms at the sides. The subject engages the butt and lifts the back off the floor, supporting with the shoulders and feet, perhaps holds for a breath or two, and brings it back down.

As far as that goes, that's fine. But, consider a moment: there are 29 vertebra in the spine. The bottom five, below the pelvis, are fused together and have very little movement. Likewise, the top two (the one connected to your skull and the one immediately below it) are also fused together. That leaves 23 joints in the spine, between the head and the hips, capable of considerable movement.

When you do the bridge as described, most of these joints move little or not at all, as the related muscles serve a primarily stabilizing role. The only considerable movement comes at the hips, shoulders and knees. Furthermore, in many cases, doing the bridge in this manner leaves too much of an arch in the lower back, which can be fine if you're standing upright, but can cause problems when your lower back is taking the stress at the center of a bridge.

Still, one may argue that, as spinal stability is a big part of the reason for this exercise, the lack of movement in most of the vertebra is a good thing. Teach them not to move, and they'll hold more steadily in practical application—that is, daily life.

I feel differently. I suggest that the more specifically one develops the joints in the vertebra and the related muscles, the better they will be at whatever task they're assigned. The more they are put through their motions, the more aware the muscles become and the greater the health benefits to them and the discs (between the vertebra), which tend to compress over time in an unaware spine, causing all kinds of pain.

Also, many people with back problems will find it difficult (painfully so) or impossible to do the bridge as described. I know. I have been one of them.

To my mind, just teaching the vertebra to hold still as a group does not lead to much individual understanding. Why not get to know them individually while using them as a group at the same time?

Starting with a variation that I learned from an excellent dance teacher, Ms. Thelma Hill, I expanded upon it to create a safer and more comprehensive format for the bridge, one beneficial to spines healthy and injured. I call it the Pelvic Curl. It has proven immensely helpful in rehabilitating my lower back, as well as the lower backs of several of my clients.

Now, let's get specific in the set-up. Yes, lie on your back. Yes, bend your knees and bring your feet toward your hips, and make a point to bring them as close to the hips as they will comfortably go.

(However, do not wiggle or lift your back to try to scoot the feet in closer. If you do, your back will not be able to move properly in the exercise. The flexibility at the knees and hips determine how far the feet come in.)

When the feet are close to the hips, the thighs get less involved, which better isolates the spine and seems to create a less stressful angle from which the lower back can work. If you are more comfortable with the legs farther out, and some people are, leave them farther out, but never with more than a 90-degree angle at the knees, as an angle greater than that can cause undue stress in the knees themselves (Photo 10).

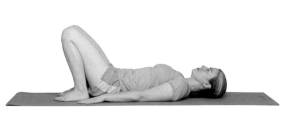

PHOTO 10

Make sure to line up your hips, knees, ankles and toes, hip-width apart, in straight lines from the hips down (Photo 11).

Be sure to keep your knees properly centered throughout the exercise and your feet forward, not turned in or out. Failing to accomplish either of these diminishes some benefits of the movement.

Place your arms, palms down, at your sides or, if you can comfortably reach them, hold your ankles, provided you don't have to strain or tug to do so.

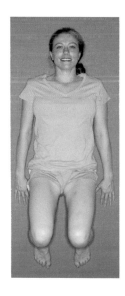

PHOTO 11

The shoulders press gently down into the body for horizontal stability and down into the floor for vertical stability, but not so far into the floor to cause any hint of an arch in the upper back.

Take a slow, deep breath. Exhale from below your navel, pressing your lower belly down into your lower spine, and your lower spine into the floor. At the same time, squeeze your butt in from the sides.

Your hips will curl upward, as if they were the blade of a shovel scooping up and away from your torso (Photo 12).

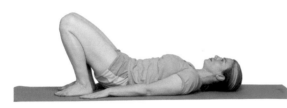

The visible movement may be very small, or fairly significant, depending on your muscular awareness, flexibility, weight and physical condition. The important thing is to learn to feel it. Don't worry about how far it moves. Find that feeling, build on that feeling, and the range of motion will come.

PHOTO 12

Some people have a hard time isolating their hips and curling them up, and instead, thinking they're doing the right thing, lift their entire backs from the upper back, relegating, once again, the bulk of their vertebra to a simple group exercise. This comes from lack of muscular sensitivity in the hips, lower belly and lower back and is remedied with a little practice.

Once you've exhaled and your hips are curled, inhale up into your rib cage, squeeze your ever-contracting lower belly down into your lower spine, and pull your butt back down to the ground. Your belly should resist uncurling throughout, but it should also lose the fight.

When the butt reaches the ground, the lower back should not be allowed to arch. Keep it flat.

Try the curl again. Use the breathing. It can help. Try at least 12 repetitions before going to the next step.

Next, we're going all the way up onto the shoulders, but not in a flat board fashion. We'll begin with the pelvic curl we just practiced, which will straighten out as the hips move into line with the knees and shoulders. Above this line, the body will begin to arch. Remember—curl below, arch above.

We'll reverse the move on the way down (which may take more practice), pulling in first with the chest and upper back before rolling down through the hips. Remember, don't go beyond what you think is safely within your capabilities.

Inhale into the ribs. As you exhale, press that lower belly into that lower back into the floor and squeeze that butt. Curl the hips slowly and powerfully upward and let them peel your back off the floor, one vertebra at a time, as they rise ever higher in steady, consecutive order. Press that belly in to hold and stabilize the curl throughout.

Keep the butt, back and belly working, keep the curling movement strong and flowing, like an ocean wave in slow, exhaling motion. One vertebra at a time. Nice and smooth.

As your upper back rises, your hips align with your knees and shoulders and that straight line is achieved (Photo 13).

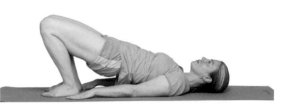

PHOTO 13

Continue the upward thrust with your hips. As the spine passes through that straight line, changing from curl to arch, press upwards through the hips and the back, especially up and through the chest, with a sense of stretching as you lift. Squeeze that belly flat against the arch and feel those muscles stabilizing the upward press of the butt, back and chest (Photo 14).

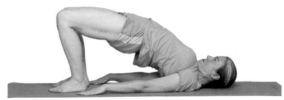

PHOTO 14

The shoulders remain stable, pressing down into the body and down into the floor. (At the top of the arch, there can be some squeezing together, in the back, of the shoulder blades for a little extra work, but that is an individual matter of safety and skill.)

If you want more, at the top of the arch, rise onto your tiptoes (Photo 15).

Lift every bit as hard in the body as you press higher through the heels and work those feet and calves.

Don't let your ankles roll open. Keep the work on the ball of the foot. (The ball of the foot is the triangle created between the big toe, the second toe, and the pad of the foot at their base.)

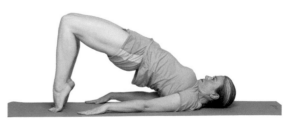

PHOTO 15

Be sure to maintain the alignment from the hips through the knees, ankles, and feet.

If you want more, squeeze your butt in a rapid (twice per second), pulsing motion, which will cause a small up and down bounce of the body. Try to pulse ever higher, with just the slightest release between pulses. Don't relax the butt too much or let it drop too far below the line of the shoulders and knees.

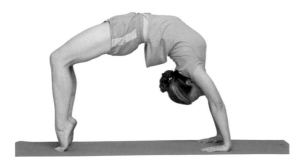

PHOTO 16

If you want more, place your palms on the floor above your shoulders and press up onto your hands and (the balls of your) feet (Photo 16).

Really lift through the body, as this position can be very stressful on the shoulders and the lower-back. If you'd like to hold the position, you must constantly press higher. If you think just to hold, your body will begin to drop ever so slightly and your joints will take all the stress. Not a good thing.

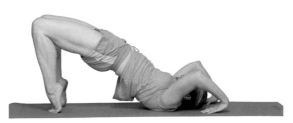

PHOTO 17

To come down, inhale deeply into your ribcage with a sense of broadening the upper back, drawing the upper abs in and under the ribs and the solar plexus (that little triangle where the ribs meet and center at the bottom of the chest) with the intake of air (Photo 17).

(If this feels too awkward, before lowering your body, bring your heels to the ground. It's easier to maneuver and easier on the back.)

With this, the chest and upper back will begin to curl in and downwards. Continue pressing up with the hips and start sucking that upper back down toward the floor, pressing the upper abs in to assist the curling (Photo 18).

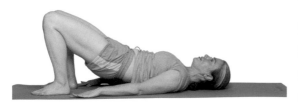

PHOTO 18

Continue to curl down through each individual vertebra. You will find your butt and lower belly have to work ever harder to sustain an upward press as the curling back descends, and the abs and middle back will be hard pressed—literally—to articulate when the downward curl reaches the middle and lower spine.

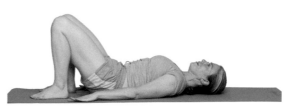

PHOTO 19

When the downward curl has run its course, the spine is again completely flat on the floor (Photo 19).

Eight repetitions should give you the idea.

SHOULDER ROTATION AND ROM

The next one is pure relaxation.

Remain on your back on the floor. Extend your knees to 90 degrees, feet flat on the floor, arms by your sides. Pull your chin in until you feel a lengthening through the back of the neck (Photo 20).

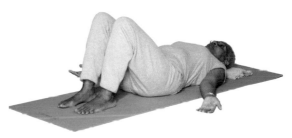

PHOTO 20

Turn your palms up and slowly sweep your arms wide, outside the body, along the floor, to the extent that your elbows remain comfortably on the floor (Photo 21).

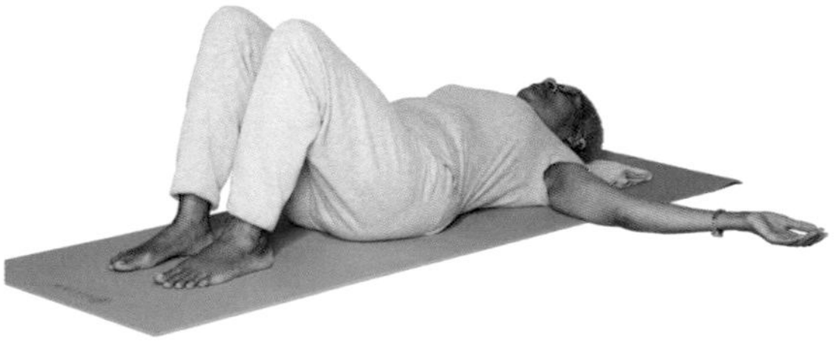

PHOTO 21

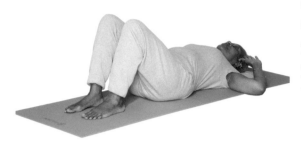

At the extent of your range, bend your elbows until the backs of your hands rest on the floor. If your shoulders are too tight to allow this, bend your elbows until the fingers are pointing toward the head (Photo 22).

PHOTO 22

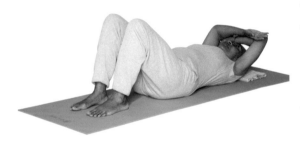

Leading with your hands, draw your arms toward the top of your head, continuing until your forearms cross each other over your forehead (Photo 23).

If it's comfortable, you may rest the arms on the floor above the head.

PHOTO 23

Resting the arms on the forehead takes the load off the (injured) shoulders and allows them to stretch safely.

If you can, continue until the left hand reaches the right elbow and the right reaches the left. Wherever the hands stop, do not grip the arms.

Let everything relax and focus on your breathing—long, deep inhales from the bottom of your belly; slow, comfy exhales from the shoulders back down.

Enjoy the stretch. Try putting the lower forearm on top. Remember to use pressure in the abs, especially the upper abs, to control the degree of arch in the spine.

To bring the arms down, stretch your legs (optional, depending on the comfort of your lower back), stretch your hands, stretch your fingers, stretch out through the elbows and slowly reach out over your head along the floor (or above it, depending on flexibility and comfort) (Photo 24).

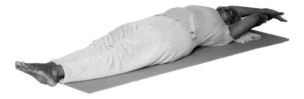

PHOTO 24

Then press wide, around and down from the top of your shoulders as you sweep your arms along the floor toward your hips (Photo 25).

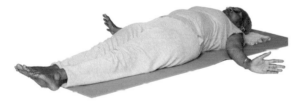

PHOTO 25

Special care should be given to the point where the arms form a Y with the body. It seems to be the point of highest stress, and there can be a feeling of the muscle rolling over the joint. There's nothing wrong with that, if it doesn't hurt, but some people find it disconcerting. (The tighter you are, the more stretch you're likely to feel. Be gentle until you gain a clear understanding.)

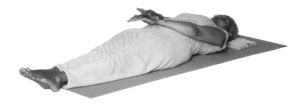

PHOTO 26

At the bottom, reach long toward the feet and lift the arms slightly to clear the legs as they cross (Photo 26) up to the elbows (full ROM), and sweep up the body, over the face and head—moving always from the shoulders (Photo 27)—to begin a second repetition reaching up and out (Photo 28).

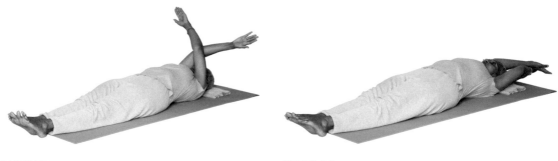

PHOTO 27   *PHOTO 28*

Be gentle, but work your entire comfortable range of motion.

After a half dozen or so repetitions, try reversing direction. Think about how the arms react in the various positions.

Be sure to maintain the shoulders securely in the body throughout the move. Don't let them rise when your arms go up. Work from the shoulder socket rather than from the neck. Work those fingers, hands and wrists to gain strength and fine-tuning.

And always, safety first.

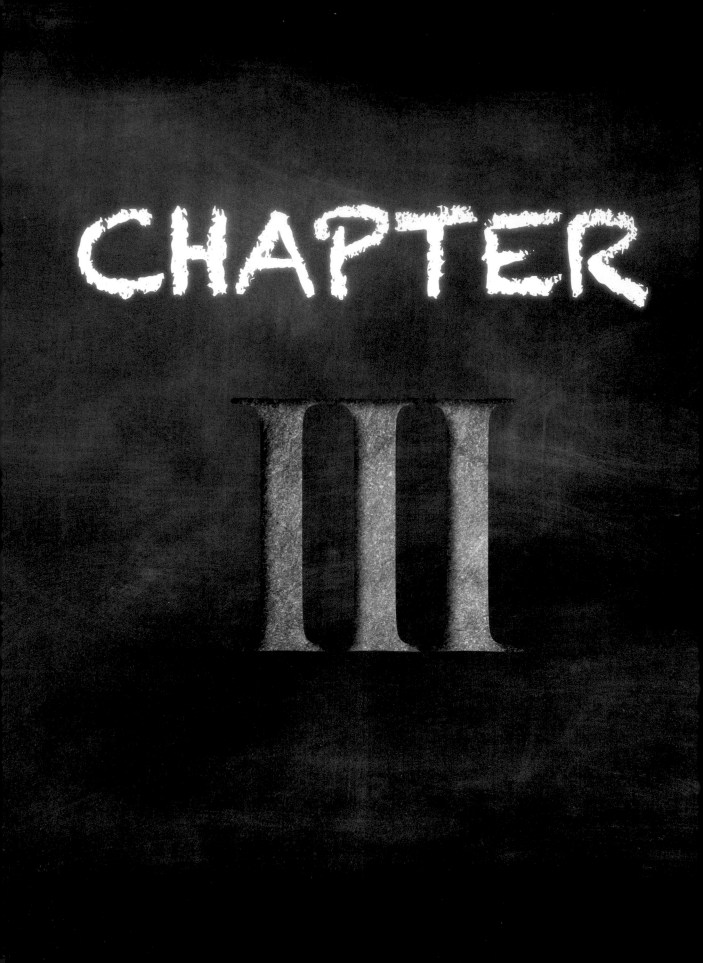

CHAPTER III: POSTURE

I use the word here defined as solid structural support for the body, whether moving or still.

THE BODY AS ARCHITECTURE

What is solid structural support? Think of a building. What keeps it standing? Solid structural support. If the weight bearing beams weren't in the right place, if the angles weren't properly aligned, if the foundation wasn't stable, a building wouldn't last very long. A little earthquake here, a little high wind there, or something as simple as too much stress on the wrong part of the building at the wrong time, and down it goes.

Have you ever stepped on an uneven surface or misjudged the drop from a curb and felt that ankle start to roll, or that knee buckle, as your body begins to fall? Same deal.

Only, buildings have it easier than us. They don't move. We do. Steel, concrete and glass have nothing to learn. Our muscles and joints do. Our support structure is not locked into place when construction is complete—for us, that's just the beginning.

If you train your muscles to properly align and support your body, they will learn. Their ability and strength will increase, and their response will become ever more automatic. On the other hand, if you ignore them, you run a high risk of degrading every aspect of your physical self and inviting sudden injury and chronic pain.

Even in the more passive activities of a sedentary lifestyle, the amount of load and stress placed on the body in the course of daily routine can be quite enough to cause all kinds of harmful complications.

An older client came to me—overweight and sedentary—with strong, chronic pain in the knees, especially in the right knee, just behind the kneecap. Almost anytime the knees were fully stretched, whether standing (supporting body weight), sitting (supporting the lower legs and feet) or lying on the back and extending the legs straight up (very little weight to support), pain was a virtual guarantee. My client told me the worst pain came when climbing stairs, which at times was nearly impossible to do.

To see for myself, I set up a couple of steps in the gym and discovered my client had a very curious way of climbing stairs that relieved the hips of their natural job of lifting the back leg and, instead, put all the force—in her case, of pulling the body forward and up—into the stepping (forward) knee and the arm pulling on the bannister, which put the point of greatest stress directly behind her forward kneecap.

We began to dedicate part of each training session to correcting the movement and the related imbalances that had come up in her body. When the proper technique was achieved, my client felt no pain climbing stairs.

So you see, even a simple movement from everyday life, repeated thousands of times over months and years, can lead to very painful bad habits and physically limiting injuries, which for many remain forever misunderstood and never fully healed.

Your body is your architecture. Build into it a solid support structure and enjoy freedom of movement, increased energy and a happier you. Let it slide, and things will creep up on you that you'll wish you'd never known.

"STAND UP STRAIGHT!"

We've all heard the words—from mothers, fathers, teachers, coaches, drill sergeants, you name it—but what do the words really mean? It sounds easy enough—

"On your feet! Tighten the legs and butt! Suck that belly in—get those shoulders back! Oh, yeah, and get that chin in..."

Yet, the fundamental thing about good posture, something I never even thought about until I was taught, is that the reason to do these things is to support your bones and your joints in a structurally sound way.

Not only does good posture protect your joints, it also teaches your muscles healthful habits and gives solid support to, and helps ensure the healthy functioning of, your internal organs. Good posture also helps protect the nerves running through every part of your body. And, believe it or not, once you learn how to stand up straight, it feels damn good.

So, let's start at the bottom and pick this thing apart.

YOUR FEET

Where should your feet be in relation to the rest of the body? All the way together? Directly under your hips? Wider than your hips? Where are your toes? Straight forward? Slightly turned out? What about your body's weight? Do you rest on your heels, your toes or both?

Most people can stand safely with their feet anywhere from twice as wide as their hips to all the way together underneath them, and there are different reasons for doing each. But, for the moment, let's keep them slightly apart, directly under the hips.

The feet can be straight forward or turned slightly open. The weight is distributed evenly on your feet from side to side, and even to slightly forward front to back. Do not sit on your heels.

YOUR KNEES

Your knees should be strong and straight, but not locked. They should line up in the same direction as the balls of your feet.

YOUR BUTT

Gently squeeze your butt from the sides in. This helps stabilize the legs and feet below to provide a solid base from which the torso can rise. Although this may make your hips rotate forward a touch, avoid curling them too far forward. Such over-rotation often occurs automatically, usually due to an unintended squeeze from underneath the butt, and inhibits the spine's ability to properly align and lift. Though this area tightens some to help stabilize the hips, until you fully understand how it feels, less may be more.

ABDOMINAL SUPPORT AND BREATHING

Next, let's talk about your belly. Your belly is an amazing thing. The "abs," as we know them, are actually just one, long muscle, in our eyes divided into a four or six or eight pack by tendons that wrap around the muscle and help contain the largely unsupported middle. Several other muscles lie around and underneath the abdominals, aiding its ability to be manipulated in so many ways. (Anyone who's ever seen a really good belly dancer ripple her belly, or a yogi do the rolling wave thing, knows what I mean.) The basic element of that ability, to be able to squeeze your belly below the navel while lifting or contracting it up and in, is easily accessible to anyone with consistent practice.

The lower abs, especially, also assist the hips in their stabilization and activate the strengthening of the lower back.

Without tucking your hips forward, gently exhale as you press your belly in below your navel. Think firm and flat. Now, keep it where it is and inhale, inward and upward, through the upper abdominal, with a sense of drawing the air and the muscles up and inside the rib cage, filling it like a sail on an old Spanish galleon.

The solar plexus, the triangle just below where the ribs join the chest, makes a good point of focus. Concentrate on an expansive feeling to the sides and a broadening of the middle of the back, rather than a great thrust forward with the middle of the chest.

THE ROLE (ROLL) OF THE SHOULDERS

Shoulders can be very troublesome things, and I will get into more detail about them later. For now, it is enough to line your shoulders up, vertically, over the highest point of your hipbone on the sides of your pelvis. The shoulders should not be rolled forward, pulled back (despite that army thing), or hunched up, but rather just pressed gently down to secure the expansion and lengthening of your torso, as well as secure the shoulders themselves. If your shoulders are habitually misaligned, pay extra attention to getting them properly set—see, think, train, adjust, and repeat as often as necessary.

THE NECK AND HEAD

That brings us to the neck and head. We all know the neck supports the head, but did you ever think of using the neck and head to lengthen the body? Lifting from the crown of your head can lighten the load on your spine, hips, knees, ankles and feet.

Look at a marionette. A string attaches at the highest point on the top of its head, pretty much in line with where its spine would be (if it had one). This is the crown of the head. Lift the string and the marionette lifts, nice and long, through the top of the head, lengthening as it lifts through the back of the neck (if it had one), leveling the chin and steadying its gaze (once again, if it had one), and standing tall.

Now, slowly relax the string and watch the marionette's body shrink and crumble. Hmmmmm.

Okay. It's time for you try it. Not the crumbling part—the standing up straight bit. But, think lifting from the top down, not pressing from the ground up.

Let's go to the mirror. (If you can't get a good full-length mirror, you might want to hire a really good mime...)

MIRROR CHECKLIST

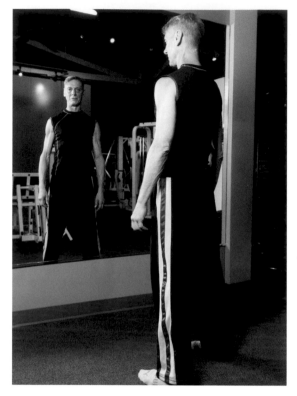

PHOTO 29

1. Are your feet together or under the hips? How is the weight distributed?

2. Looking down, are your knees aiming in the same direction as the balls of your feet? Knees should be straight, but not locked.

3. Squeeze your butt. Does your pelvis rotate forward? A little is fine, but not too much. Your lower spine should retain a natural curve.

4. Take a big breath and exhale, pressing in below the navel.

5. Inhale deeply up under the rib cage. Feel that broadening in the chest and middle of the back as you grow taller through the spine. Keep that expansive, tall feeling as you exhale.

6. Inhale again and lift through the crown of the head, lengthening the back of the neck and leveling the chin. Press your shoulders down gently, at the same time, to stabilize the lift of the torso (Photo 29).

7. Now, turn profile to the mirror and try it all again.

THINGS TO CONSIDER— TROUBLESHOOTING

THE FEET

If you're having trouble distributing your weight evenly to the insides and outsides of your feet, check the following.

If the weight is primarily on the insides of your feet:

1. You may have flat feet (fallen arches).

2. You may have alignment problems from the knees and hips.

3. You may have weakness or imbalances in the muscles of the legs and feet.

To check your arches, take off your shoes and turn the inside of your foot to the mirror. Does the space between the heel and the ball of the foot have an upward curve or a downward curve? Is the outside edge of the foot in this area lifted somewhat or flat to the ground? If the arch is normal, it should appear lifted with an upward curve.

Flat feet can allow an overly outward rotation of the ankle, which can cause problems to muscles and joints up through your body. If you have any concerns, see an orthopedist. Both flat feet and high arches can benefit from arch supports in the shoes, as well as certain types of exercise we will discuss later.

THE KNEES

To check the alignment of the knees, stand facing the mirror and put your legs together. Do the feet come together, or is there a space between them? The feet, in this position, will come together if your knees are straight or bowed. If the knees touch, but the feet don't, you knees are somewhat "knocked."

Optimally, one should be able to draw a straight, vertical line from the hips through the knees to the balls of the feet. Having said that, let me point out that, if, in my whole life, I've seen three people with legs that have grown perfectly straight, that's all I've seen. It's very rare. Generally, we're all a little bent.

Personally, I got me some bowed legs.

If you carry the weight of your body more on the outsides of your feet, you are probably a bit bow-legged as well. Many of us are, and it tends to encourage an inward rotation of the feet. In the mirror, the feet will come together, but there will be an outward curve to the legs and the space between them will be widest at the knees.

One way to get an idea about your ankles' alignment is to look at the heels of your shoes. Are they worn evenly down the middle or more to one side or the other? This is a good indication of your habitual weight distribution, which does have an impact on the muscular balance of your legs and hips.

While the rotation of the ankles can generally be modified considerably with focused exercises and constant vigilance, the same is not necessarily true of the knees. Those who are knock-kneed, and the bowlegged among us, are, to some extent, stuck with what we've got, especially if our bones have finished growing. Once the knee joints are set in their tracks, realigning the knees is something that may be possible, but must, to my mind, be approached cautiously and with an eye to a commitment of several months, at the very least, before there will be any noticeable change. The last thing you want to do is cause pain, instability and tracking problems in your knees.

A safer, and more doable, idea would be to maintain the legs as they are and not allow them to knock or bow any farther. That is, of course, if "as they are" is a healthy place to be. If one's legs are so far bowed or knocked that one or more joints is constantly being pressured in a harmful way, the situation must be relieved.

If your knees, when bent, will not line up with the balls of your feet, you've got a rotational problem. To find out, stand with your feet under your hips, keep your weight in your heels and bend your knees a bit, no more than 90 degrees. Do not put your weight on your toes or allow your knees to go past the end of your toes.

As you bend, keep your knees in line with the balls of your feet. (Do not put your weight on your toes or allow your knees to go past the end of the toes.) If this is difficult or painful, you've got a problem.

If the problem is muscle awareness, a remedy can be easily found. However, if the bones in the joint have grown into this line of tracking, any work to correct it must be done slowly and cautiously, and successful maintenance might be a better alternative.

THE HIPS

The structure of the hips can also be a culprit when it comes to the tracking and alignment of the knees and feet.

Some people have a particularly narrow pelvis, which can have an adverse effect on the lower limbs (and the lower back). Others have a pelvis that curves slightly in from the sides, rotating the bone structure of the hip sockets somewhat inwardly, which also can cause problems in the knees.

Both of these things are difficult, if at all possible, to improve. Nevertheless, a healthy way of controlling these situations can usually be found.

A much easier alignment problem to correct, in this part of the body, is purely in the way you move your legs. Work from the hips down, control your thighs and knees, align them properly with the ankles and feet. Don't just follow from the ground up.

THE ABDOMINALS

Don't be surprised if you have a hard time getting your belly to do what you want at first. You'll get there. As you get to know your muscles better, they will get better at serving you.

In terms of feeling them work specifically, that can take longer. Be patient, do the work. Build them, and they will hum.

THE BACK

It's generally easier to see what's going on with the back in profile. Regarding posture, there are two common ways of carrying oneself that are thoughtlessly destructive:

1. The lower spine overarches forward (usually accompanied by a loose lower belly). To compensate (maintain balance), some people overarch the upper body to the back, lifting the front of the rib cage and drawing the shoulders back above the protruding butt, giving a tall visual impression at an unaffordable price.

   Others will collapse the bottom of the chest, letting the middle of the torso push back to balance above the butt. This move is accompanied by shoulders that roll forward, hunching the upper back and crunching the bones in the neck as the chin pokes forward.

2. This same upper-body collapse will also accompany the second standard lower spine misalignment, that of tucking the hips forward and flattening the lower back. However, in this case, the middle back remains above the flat lower back, and the hips and shoulders roll forward to balance the body.

Either of these approaches are high risk for immediate, lingering and long-term pain. Correcting them can take time, as the muscles are often quite attached to their bad habits.

THE SHOULDERS

That definitely holds true for the shoulders. They are often among the least aware groups of muscles, as there are so many different things we can do with them.

I think the people with the hardest time are those who have habitually let their shoulders roll forward. Their awareness of their rhomboid muscles—the guys that pull the shoulder blades together into the middle of the back—is usually extremely poor and takes quite some time to develop.

For those who overarch their upper back, it's more the reverse—learn to relax the rhomboids a bit and support through the upper abs into the solar plexus, broadening the middle back and bringing the ribcage in line while pressing in through the lower belly.

Poor shoulder alignment causes all kinds of pain, from the blades on up into the neck, and, in certain cases, down into the arms, hands and fingers.

THE NECK

Yes, the neck. Most of its problems, barring accidents, come from everything below. The posture of the rest of your body very much determines the comfort and alignment of your neck. Get that posture together, learn to lift from the top of your head, use the range of motion in your neck regularly, and you'll be fine.

Another villain is tension. Many of us carry tension in our necks and shoulders. Part of letting that tension go comes with correcting posture. More specific remedies can be found in the next three chapters.

CHAPTER

IV

CHAPTER IV: EXERCISE

WHY

If you tried the exercises in the previous chapter (and, yes, stretches done properly are exercise), I'd be willing to bet at least some part of them felt good as you did them, or you felt better after doing them.

That's the point. Or at least a big part of it. A properly working body works better; a properly working body feels better. Take care of your body, and it will take care of you. Don't, and live out your life in a cumbersome, unstable and ever more limiting machine, with a perpetually increasing risk of malfunction and pain.

Speaking of which, many of the older or more sedentary who try the Reclining Overhead Stretch through the shoulders' range of motion (chapter II, Photos 20-28) will find not only some aches and groans along the way, but also a limited ability to reach overhead.

The reasons for this are good examples of what happens when you don't maintain your body:

1. If you don't regularly use the full ROM in your shoulders, it will get smaller. If it's not in your workout and it's not in your daily life, you're not regularly using it.

    "If you don't use it, you _____ it." (fill in the blank)

2. Ignoring your shoulders' ROM often leads to, or comes with, a rolling forward of the upper body as the chest tightens and the back relaxes. As this bad habit settles in, the neck and the muscles that reach out from it to the shoulders are stressed in potentially painful ways.

The result—habitually poor alignment with limited ability in the neck, shoulders and upper back, almost certainly chronic pain in one or all of these areas, and an upper spine hunching, invisibly, a little more every day, day by day, week in, month out, year after year, until one morning you look in the mirror and wonder what happened to that tall, vibrant you that now exists only in your memory and any surviving photographs.

You may not figure out exactly how it happened, but I guarantee you'll have a hunch.

Everything that exists, us included, is constantly changing. For our bodies, for our lives, these changes come in two sizes—better and worse.

There is no staying the same. Grow actively or grow old.

WHAT'S YOUR PLEASURE?

Everyone who looks for an exercise program wants something safe and effective. That's great, but don't stop there. Find something that inspires you.

It can be hard enough to get off your duff and out the door to go work out when you know that, once you've warmed up, you'll enjoy doing what you're doing. But, to get up extra early in the morning, or finally get home after a long day and try to stay motivated before you're too settled in—that can become impossible when you know you won't like what lies ahead. Even if you do push through uninspiring exercise for a time, your chances of sticking with it for the long term are poor at best.

So find something you like. Find something you'll enjoy sticking with.

I'm a skills guy myself—it started with sports as a kid. I was fascinated with almost everything that came along, and I played a lot of ball, especially baseball and football, for years.

In and out of college, I moved on to fencing and dance. I was lucky in fencing—being left-handed turned out to be a huge advantage. It really shook people up, though I've never quite figured out why.

Dance, on the other hand, was extremely demanding. It took a very long time to become anywhere near good—I often felt like an idiot—but, once it felt right—when the power, speed, control and precision at last came together and I could cut loose—that was a blast!

The most recent addition to my training came as a natural extension of my years living in New York. In the City I found myself, from time to time, in situations requiring physical defense. For the safety of all concerned (myself and other innocents especially), I began studying martial arts, which, as it turns out, I really, really love.

The point is, there's something for each individual body and every personality, and that includes you.

Maybe you like sports. These days, there are untold numbers to choose from. Sports can improve your coordination, dexterity, bone strength, joint strength, muscle strength, flexibility, your cardiovascular (heart, blood vessels and lungs) system and improve both your efficiency and rate of digestion. Not to mention turn fat into muscle and, if you wish, burn that fat off entirely and lose weight.

Maybe you're like me, drawn to the physical disciplines—acrobatics, dance, gymnastics, martial arts, yoga. There are easier and tougher, softer and harder styles within all of these. Their benefits can include all those found in sports, as well as a much more finely tuned body, which will bring you considerable insight into the way you move through your daily life. There are practical applications for what you've learned, as well—at least with martial arts and yoga.

Maybe you want to lift weights, put on some size and rip it up. That's great! Just do it right. Don't get too tight (watch your flexibility) and lay off the steroids! Building lean mass means stronger muscles, bones and joints and an improved digestive system, not to mention a physique that will be admired by many. There can also be, if you wish, cardiovascular gains to be made through lifting weights.

Whatever your pleasure, if it's been a while, you may want to start off easy. Learn to manage any chronic pain; fix alignment, strength, and flexibility imbalances; and find safe exercises that burn off weight without jeopardizing the joints. Help for all such issues can be found in the various forms of exercise presented in the last chapter.

So, pick whatever you like. If your first choice doesn't work out, try different things until something gets you.

Having a body that knows how to move, that knows how to react (although no body's perfect and dumb accidents do happen), a body that brings freedom, energy and enthusiasm to your life is a wonderful thing. It's part of you being you at your best.

My question is, why be anything else?

WHAT TO EXPECT

Although different types of exercise bring different rewards, there are a few that apply across the board.

HEAVY BREATHING

With the exception of yoga and tai chi, which emphasize deep, slow, even breathing, any exercise regimen requiring regular exertion should leave you huffing and puffing, at least from time to time.

That's a good thing. Pushing yourself beyond what you're accustomed to is what builds strength, flexibility and, in this case, endurance. When you're breathing hard, you're benefiting your heart, lungs and circulatory system.

Having said that, there are two different ways of huffing and puffing.

Aerobic: In *aerobic* (more commonly known as "cardio") exercise, oxygen is used in the process of creating energy for the body, in much the same way as oxygen feeds the fire in a furnace. Oxygen is not the fuel but, without it, the fuel could not burn. (Fat will be involved, too, but oxygen is the grease—in this case—that turns the wheel.)

As you increase your speed or intensity, it becomes ever harder for your oxygen-based energy conversion system, which can only burn so fast, to keep up. That's when you body goes:

Anaerobic: If you work hard enough, you push past your aerobic limit. To get all you've got left to give, your body dips into fuel reserves in your cells. At this point, you shift from *aerobic* to *anaerobic* (without oxygen) exercise.

Good news is, in anaerobic mode, you can fly like the wind, leap like a lizard or train like Jake Fury. Pity of it is, you've only got about two minutes before you run out of gas.

(*Anaerobic* exercise is a term used to differentiate from *aerobic* exercise. It does not mean your oxygen supplied system ceases to produce when you're past your aerobic limit. Anaerobic actually only describes the extra bit of energy production. You're still using oxygen at maximum levels throughout.)

It is good to train in both these methods of energy production. Each enhances the other, though regular work in either can lead to cardiovascular improvement. Still, you've got to be ready for them.

Food must also be considered. Some people feel better with a little food in their bellies before their exercise, others don't. If you do eat, keep it light and lean; those who eat seem to fare best with whole grains, yogurt, fruits, juices, smoothies—that sort of thing. Only you can know best what works for you.

If you're already into heavy breathing, you've probably come to know the boundaries of your aerobic and anaerobic abilities well, and how you feel when you reach them. If you're relatively new, you might want to take it a little easy at first.

It is not uncommon for unconditioned runners to get seriously nauseous when they push too hard on a relatively long run, or for new martial arts students to throw in more than the towel after a few rounds of sparring. Such things are neither fun nor necessary.

However, newness to exercise should never be used as an excuse to limit your work to what is comfortable. Comfortable will not get you there. Comfortable, if anything, is part of the problem.

Let's say you're new to running. Yes, you should take it a little easier until you see how your body reacts. After that, to my mind, if you can carry on a steady conversation while you're running, you're not running hard enough. You should at least push yourself near the edge of discomfort.

Same goes with lifting weights, calisthenics—anything. If you don't work hard, your results will disappoint you. No challenge. No victory. No reward.

So, get out of breath. See what it's like. Try that two minutes to failure thing (anaerobic). Take a run, as fast as you can, for 20 minutes or so (aerobic). Learn to huff. Learn to puff. And don't forget to smile.

THE PAINFUL TRUTH

I'm going to give it to you straight. Exercise, done properly, will make you sore. (That should take that smile off your face.) If you're new, if you're trying something new, if you stick with your regular routine and work to your limit, soreness will be thine.

If it's the right kind of soreness, that's a good thing. If it's the wrong kind of pain, measures must be taken.

The right kind of soreness will be muscle soreness. In the areas affected, the muscles will feel sore to the touch and tight, especially near the joints, whose comfortable ROM will be smaller.

The wrong kind of pain comes in several flavors. It can be sharp as an electric shock; it can burn like spreading fire; it can jerk tight like a piece of overstretched rope. It can be a dull or rhythmical ache that haunts you when you rest, but disappears once you warm up. It's pretty much anything that isn't (only) muscle stiffness and soreness.

An injury can hit you so fast that your body will have reacted before you know you're hurt. Or an injury might wait for hours, even overnight, to show itself, creeping up on you slowly while you're at rest.

Injuries can neither be ignored nor toughed out without making them worse. They must be cared for as soon as they occur. Seek professional assistance, ask questions, read chapter IX: **Injury and Recovery**.

Having said that, muscle soreness itself can be a serious drag when taken too far. If you wake up the next day and your muscles are a bit sore to the touch and there's some stiffness in the joints, that's fine. It actually can feel good once you get moving. You know you've had a meaningful workout, and the soreness advances your physical sensitivity.

On the other hand, it is possible to work out so hard (especially with heavy weights) that the next day there's no soreness at all. Nor the day after that. Maybe not even the third day.

But, on the fourth day, or the fifth day, you wake up to a body that can barely be moved. You lie there bewildered, aching just to be still, hopelessly imprisoned by the agonizing concretions of your once supple muscles that surround and now bind your joints in torturous stiffness. (Think Baron von Frankenstein's favorite boy burning in the fire.)

I do not exaggerate the degree of soreness that accompanies this phenomenon. Lifting a coffee cup, turning a steering wheel—these can become major operations. If that isn't bad enough, the effect of extreme muscle soreness takes about as many days to go away as it does to come on.

The extent to which one experiences these particular pleasures of the flesh is a matter of personal experience, choice and philosophy. Some people will eagerly seek the extremes, others feel a little goes a long way.

However sore you want to be, whether you choose a softer or harder route, health and safety make a good bottom line.

IS THREE ENOUGH? IS SIX TOO MANY?

Estimates for the minimum weekly amount of exercise required to maintain or improve one's health vary from a low of 20 minutes, three times a week, to as much as one hour every day of at least moderate intensity.

All I can say about that low end is, it would have to be a 20-minute freight train at full throttle to even hope to see any real results, and I still don't think you'd get much. Plus, to burn that hard without really warming up (there wouldn't be time), you'd have to be in pretty incredible shape, which you wouldn't be if you only did three 20-minute sessions a week.

(I must point out, however, that in the case of severe injuries or long-term, chronic debilitation, 20 minutes three times a week, or 10 minutes each day, at a low to moderate intensity, might actually become a goal to reach for in the beginning weeks of recovery.)

Still, my teachers always taught, and medical research has continued to support the idea, that yes, only three times a week is required for minimum healthy physical training.

Even so, I believe my teachers would have laughed at the presumed adequacy of 20-minute sessions (their classes ran one-and-a-half to three hours, and there was nothing moderate about them). Nor would they have recommended only three days a week to a healthy student. Invariably, they all encouraged training either six or seven days a week.

(For myself, it has become clear over the years that I require a bare minimum of one good hour, three times a week, to even have a shot at keeping my body healthy. Less than that leaves me exposed to a severe spinal defect that I can only manage with regular exercise.

That doesn't mean that my body's happy with only three days a week. It's just the least I can do and stay healthy.)

So, three days a week minimum. Three minimum—and make them count. Push yourself. Focus exclusively on your exercise and work at a reasonably tough intensity. Don't break your rhythm, don't stop and chat. If you have been more sedentary, you will begin to show improvement. If you have been more active, you will at least provide baseline maintenance for your body—much better than nothing, though your edge will dull a bit.

A rumor that has long circulated around gyms is that training every day is bad for you. I think training daily is actually optimal, excepting certain body-building regimens, as long as you know what you're doing and respect your limits.

If you're learning skills, you'll be amazed how much more rapidly you progress when training every day. Pursuing skill or not, your body will transform much more quickly as well.

(Overtraining, which may be one origin of this rumor, is something else entirely. As the name implies, you're overdoing it. Overtraining occurs when your rest and nutrition are inadequate to the intensity and duration of your daily workouts.)

Balance. It's always needed.

If you're new to exercise, and you can't make it every day, try every other day. It's much easier to stay motivated working out every other day than three days a week.

The problem with three days a week is that it comes with two days off in a row, which tickle your comfort zone with a great temptation to take off a third. When you take that third day off, a fourth is even easier to justify. Then it's five, six, next week...next month...dum dum d'dum daah d'dum d'dum d'dum.

It's much easier to get in a healthy rhythm on an every other day schedule. Wait until your body is enthused and working out regularly before you tempt it with too much couch.

VISUAL EYES

People often want to know how long it takes to see results. On the obvious end, the harder you work, the sooner you see them. But that's only part of the story.

Diet plays a huge role. You must supply your body with the nutrition it needs. Heavily processed food and foods overloaded with fats, sugar and salt (often the same animal) will not get you where you want to go. And remember how calories work: burn more than you consume = lose weight; consume more than you burn – gain weight.

With a healthy diet, a good exercise program and good exercise form, many encouraging signs will appear rather quickly. Even working out only three days, one hour each per week—if they're good hours—you'll start to feel better within a couple of weeks and look better within a month. At five days or more, one hour each, obvious visual changes—less jiggle, more contour in the arms, a shrinking waistline, firmer backside and thighs—show up in as little as 10 days.

However, to really wake your muscles up, to get to know them individually and have them respond with automatic precision, takes longer. In the smaller muscle groups, many of the finer movements needed for sports and physical disciplines can take years to refine.

But don't worry. Large muscle groups, and the more basic aspects of the smaller, can, with steady work, be at your bidding in as little as six weeks (time varies by individual).

When running an outdoor, five-day, six-week boot camp program, I came across a boot camper who, obsessed with her waistline, constantly complained that, regardless of how much lower belly work we did, she never felt anything.

On the last day, the thirtieth session, as I put the campers through their last lower belly ordeal, she suddenly shrieked, "I feel it!"

She screamed so loudly, I thought she was injured. I rushed to her side. "What? What are you feeling?"

"I feel my lower belly!" she cried. Her lower belly sensitivity had just kicked in. I was so relieved I laughed out loud. She was ecstatic.

She was now equipped with a key element necessary to support her body healthfully for the rest of her life.

Obvious visual changes in body contour (growing lean muscle and burning off fat) show up pretty fast. Coordinative skills—the muscle sensitivity required to change bad habits, correct posture, develop a solid core and refine movement—depends on where you're starting from and how far you want to go, but can take a considerable amount of time.

Never get discouraged. Just do the work. The results will come.

ONE MESA TROUBLE

If you have been dedicated to maintaining your body or improving your physical skills for more than a year, and you've been working very hard at it, you may have encountered what many call a "plateau," a level of development that, no matter how hard you try, you don't seem to improve beyond.

Don't worry about it. There's a natural reason for plateaus, and there are ways to continue your climb.

Plateaus have both physical and psychological causes.

In my experience, there are three primary reasons why you plateau physically.

1. The first is that muscles become more efficient in the movements and exercises they regularly do. The more efficiently they work, the less energy they burn in the movement and, if you're looking for size, the harder you must push to make any gains. There may come a time when your muscles and joints will reach the limit of stress they can safely endure in such situations.
    A good strategy is to alter the exercise while still working the same muscle(s). It doesn't take a huge change in movement to bring muscles to a less efficient place where they must again work harder, and there are several ways to do so. Alter the angle, alter the weight, alter the ROM.
    Think of it as a fresh approach. Later, when they're no longer routine, you can return to the abandoned versions of the exercises, if you wish, and the challenge they once gave you should be renewed.
    Changing the way the muscles are challenged will also have an effect on how the muscles sculpt. Consider, if you will, the human butt. It will form differently built on in-line skates than it will built on running; it will form differently built by a ballerina than a martial artist.
    When choosing your exercise, a little forethought for your backside—and other body parts—may give you more of what you're looking for. Think of it as evolution by intelligent design.

2. The second reason, related to the first, applies more to competitive sports and the physical disciplines.

    When you train daily, or almost daily, as hard as you can, there will be periods of an apparent lack of progress. You can't improve your speed, can't gain any height in that jump, still can't get through that combination and keep your balance. What's a mother to do?

A few things:

A) First, re-examine your technique. There is a streamline for everything, a perfect way for your body to execute any move, and you can make it or break it by centimeters, maybe even millimeters.

    A dancer might achieve a challenging, whole-body movement with nothing more than a quarter-inch adjustment to a shoulder. A runner might find that the least little lift in the chest makes all the difference for breath and speed. An acrobat might hit or miss a mark from nothing more than the angle of the elbow or the position of the chin, something easily overlooked in the overall crunch of intensive training.

    So, be precise. Re-evaluate your technique. The central part of the movement may have nothing to do with your inability to perfect it. Poke around. Micromanage. No one else can do it for you to the extent that you can do it for yourself.

B) Second, you may want to try cross-training, working the same muscles toward the same goal in new and different ways. Distance runners (endurance cardio) may want to go anaerobic for a while and burn hot and fast to exhaustion (running sprints/stairs/hills). Such work can actually improve their endurance. A swimmer might spend more time working out of the water, instead of in it, building the same strengths.

    Cross-training can snap your muscles out of any routine-induced trance into which they may have fallen, and give your eyes renewed perspective on the prize.

    Even in the physical disciplines, their can be times when cross-training is the best option available. When I was too injured to dance, but my large muscle groups were intact, I ran for three months. It was easy after years of intense, anaerobic work in the classroom. I started at 2.2 miles on flat terrain and quickly progressed to over four.

    Returning to class three months later, I danced better than I had when I left. My movement had more freedom, my mind was refreshed, and my feet were planted firmly on that next, higher plateau.

C) There is one more physical factor, in at least some of these situations, which, perhaps, is never fully considered. That factor is the way our muscles learn.

Studying for years in the same techniques, it's become clear to me that plateaus are a natural and normal part of physical progress. When training one's body in detail, trying to perfect tiny and precise movements and huge and explosive movements, it seems the muscles often need considerable time growing into all that fine-tuning before they are capable of taking the next step. There is a learning absorption process, a "soaking in" of information, as it has been described in martial arts, in which time requirements vary for each individual.

From my experience, I have come to believe that all forms of exercise follow some variation of this theme. Often during this process, the outward signs of improvement may be few to none, but that doesn't mean your body isn't getting ready to make that next big jump.

3. The third physical reason one might plateau is simple—insufficient nutrition.

When I first began lifting weights, I continually grew stronger, but my body didn't change. I thought about it for a while and, after six months, I decided to increase my intake of healthy foods and calories.

My muscles began to grow, the bit of fat at my sides thinned, my waist trimmed, my shoulders filled out. Though I gained a few pounds, my waist became both leaner and more streamlined than it had been before. I also had considerably more energy.

That made me realize how foolishly I'd worried about eating too much as a dancer, from a misguided concern to maintain a long and lean physique. Weight was never a problem for me—I was active all day long—but energy sometimes had been.

I surmised then that a lack of sufficient nutrition had been the reason why, often in the fourth or fifth hour of class or rehearsal, my butt would be dragging when it seemed the other dancers' butts were still riding high. (Not that I let anyone else notice, but, internally, it was sometimes quite a struggle.)

If I'd eaten adequately, my energy would've been higher, and I bet I would've had a stronger, leaner and meaner—in the best possible sense of the term—physique.

So eat enough and of the right stuff.

The psychological aspect of training—how you focus and how you think—can strand you on a plateau for far longer than your muscles' learning curve ever could. You can become so involved with all the things you need to get right to perfect your moves that your thinking becomes an obstacle to your progress. You won't see the forest for the trees.

The insidious nature of this nasty cerebral affliction increases in direct proportion to the level of skill you strive to achieve. The more technical the work, the more thoughts you have to untangle.

Even in simple calisthenics, those with uneducated structural or coordinative skills can struggle just to get basic exercise form right. If it takes too long, they may cross that fine line between hope and despair. At that point, the idea of "I'll never get it right!" easily becomes the new boundary of their ability and, every time one of those things they think they can't do comes up, they lose their focus, prove themselves right and perform the exercise poorly.

If you're stuck in such a hole but your form, perfect or not, is not harmful to your structure, you can, if you wish, accept your limitation, though it will have an effect on how you develop.

On the other hand, if you wish to get past it, I know of two options: one you must consciously choose, and one that may be thrust upon you. They both amount to the same thing—getting over your stigma, getting past your mental block.

The first is to conscientiously back off, mentally and emotionally. Accept that it's going to take time. Let go of your frustration (I always feel frustrated when I hear that). Frustration is a distraction. It's not what you're there for.

Keep working, but develop patience. Yes, **develop** patience. Patience is seldom adequately supplied just for the asking.

Let it be okay to screw up. Practice steadily and without prejudice. You'll get there.

The other option is to change everything for a week or so, do something completely different, get entirely away from your routine. This will allow not only your mind to relax, but also your muscles will get some relative rest and relaxation as well. All that technical stuff you've been studying will have a chance to soak deeper into your body and drain out of the front of your mind. After a few days, when you get back to it, you'll be surprised to find your skill has magically improved.

Sometimes, though, when you don't feel you're making progress, stubbornness can arise, a refusal to let up. You determine to relentlessly move forward and let nothing stop you.

Sometimes that works. Sometimes, you break through that barrier and it's all sunshine and roses. Sometimes, your body goes on strike. That's where that "thrust upon you" bit I mentioned comes in.

Short-term injuries—those that force you to take a few days or a week off, though always a drag and an apparent interruption of your progress can, as strange as it sounds, actually be a blessing.

Mentally, a forced pause in your training serves a double purpose. You may not get past your frustration, but it will no longer be focused on your skill. You'll be thinking about pain, about getting past that injury, about feeling normal again. Less immediate frustrations will fade. You may even come to the point of accepting the situation—then everything calms down.

A short-term injury will also remind you how nice it is to feel healthy, free to pursue your goals, without keeping you away from those pursuits for too long. Concern over your skill level diminishes considerably against the excitement of recovering and feeling good again, getting back to training.

When you are ready to begin again, your new attitude will make a huge difference. At least for a few days, you'll forget to nag yourself about your shortcomings, and they will begin to file out the door.

FORM, BABY, FORM

Although the reasons people give for exercising are many, virtually all of them are tied to looking better and feeling better. We want to get leaner, have more energy, fit that hot new bikini (except for most guys on that last one). We want to like what we see in the mirror.

But for the injured and skill seeking, few ever cite improving their form (body support and mechanics) as a primary goal. Yet, form is what drives posture and movement (not to mention how the muscles develop). What's the point of being well sculpted if you're trapped in bad posture and limited in agility?

Form is a deceptively small word for all that it implies:

1. The general position of the legs, arms and torso

2. The finer alignments of the torso, limbs, hands, feet, neck and head

3. How the muscles are used

4. How breathing is involved

5. The degree to which one can recognize and release—search and destroy—unnecessary tension in the body (squeezing the lips or the corners of the mouth, tightening the jaw, the forehead, neck or shoulders, gripping the fingers or toes)

6. One's ability to perform movement in a strong, fluid, controlled manner

All of these things are necessary to get the best and safest out of your work. Pity of it is, most of us don't see past number 1. I guess most of us assume that, if we get the general movement right, that's good enough.

I beg to differ. Consider the traditional push-up. Almost everyone gets the bending of the elbows as the obvious movement and, achieving this, thinks the job accomplished. Yet, upon reviewing the overall structure, we find some very interesting curiosities.

As the arms bend, some people drop their heads down, poking their noses to the ground. As the arms stretch, some slack their bellies and sway their backs, breaching like whales from the water, upper bodies rising while their lower bodies drag on the floor. Throughout the movement, different people may have their faces distorted, shoulders hunched, chests protruded, butts pushed heavenward—the possibilities are endless. The complications that arise from these distorted visions can be endless as well.

When such aberrations need correcting, as do all those mentioned, yet they remain unaddressed, they grow worse. Eventually, a body that once held such promise can end up looking more like the renowned and repugnant historic bell ringer of a certain cathedral in Paris. That's a high price for fame.

The thing is, everything you want to achieve in physical fitness begins with good form. From the most precise pitcher of 101-mph fastballs to the most basic squatter or lifter of weights, there is at least one right way and any number of wrong ways to perform any movement. Get it wrong and suffer; get it right and thrive.

I admit the idea of perfecting form is not a very sexy one. But, as I said before, leave your ego at home. Get your form together first—sexy will naturally follow. Once you've thoroughly educated your mind and developed your eye and your muscular awareness; when you've examined all the different parts of your structure individually, through various movements, and put them together as a whole and found them sound, then all good things will lie within your grasp.

You'll be able to throw those heavy weights around while a cute babe's watching, and she'll admire not only your muscles but your form as well, and you won't be hurting yourself in the bargain. You can feed your internal Amazon with fierce punches and kicks that split the air like thunder, without jeopardizing your joints. You can let your thoughts melt away as your body moves in the more subliminal rhythms that flow spontaneously from years of rigorous, conscious training, all the while increasing your chances for a long, healthy, active and pain-free life.

So, while you're exercising, rather than routinely going through the motions, why not use the opportunity to review your technique and correct any bad structural habits?

Break it down. Is the primary force for the move supplied by the muscles you're trying to work? If you're working your shoulders, are you moving from your shoulders (we tend to move from our hands)? Could there be a better angle for the same move?

Are the supporting joints safely aligned or are one or more of them being unnecessarily stressed? What's the rest of the body up to? What about your belly? Where's the weight on your feet? Even lying on a bench, pressing weights, the entire body has a supporting role to play.

Remember, form requires time. Form requires patience. Form requires deep and thorough examination.

Train your eye. You can't correct what you can't see. Train your body. You can't control what you can't feel. Train your mind. You can't fix what you don't know is broken.

IN THE CLASSROOM

Just as we take classes for different reasons, there are different reasons for the ways classes are taught. The first two exemplify the differences between studying in a facility dedicated to learning a physical skill versus the same skill-type class taught in a commercial fitness center.

1. In a facility dedicated to learning a skill, the focus is on form and technique. The intensity of the workout is secondary to achieving technical goals.
   In a fitness center, the focus is on giving you a good workout.

2. In the first, one devotes years to steady training.
   In the second, you go when you want; you don't when you don't want.

3. In the first, the teacher will verbally define, or demonstrate, or have a senior student demonstrate, the exercise, then the students will perform it as the teacher observes and corrects their technique. A brief pause often occurs between exercises.
   In the second, the teacher usually performs the moves along with the students. There is a constant flow to the work being done. As both the students and teachers must observe and perform at the same time, some technical considerations fall by the wayside.

4. In the first, the demands on the muscles and joints become ever more precise as the level of difficulty increases. These demands cannot be ably (or, often, safely) approached without having done, and continuing to do, thousands of repetitions of more basic technical training, under the scrutinizing eye of a teacher.

    In the second, though there are more and less difficult movements, they all remain (though not necessarily safely) within the grasp of your average newbie. The teacher tries to keep an eye on everyone but—once again—the teacher is working, too.

    Don't get me wrong. Any good instructor at a fitness center will, throughout the class, give constant verbal pointers and corrections. But the instructor must also, at the same time, perform the exercises physically and cue the movements vocally, both of which require a considerable degree of concentration. Only occasionally do such instructors find the chance to focus all of their attention purely on the students. Because of this, the opportunity to truly learn form and technique remains diminished.

5. In the first, as one's skill improves, one advances by class level—basic, beginner, intermediate, advanced, professional (often only with the permission of, or an invitation from, the teacher)—or some other form of acknowledged advancement, such as the belt system in many martial arts. Depending on one's drive and ability, the sky's the limit for what can be learned.

    In fitness centers, virtually all classes are open to anyone wishing to take them. Though there is often plenty of room for a student to improve within this format, the level of skill that can be acquired remains limited.

6. For those who study skills, there is always further to go. Perfection can never be (consistently) maintained and must be constantly pursued. Training is concentrated on the skills being studied. In a fitness center, though some level of skill can be acquired, any deep understanding will probably need to be looked for elsewhere. Most who take classes use them as part of a broader weekly exercise routine and have no intention of pursuing the skills involved more seriously.

7. In a dedicated facility, if you don't take it seriously, you may not be there very long. Teachers of competitive and professional skills often have little patience for students who give less than their best, feeling they waste the class's time. Even a dedicated student may get a harsh phrase or ten if the teacher feels they're slacking.

    Instructors in fitness centers tend to be nice, energetic, encouraging, motivating and sympathetic at all times (unless the format of the class requires some (role-playing) tough talk—as in a boot camp).

So, the idea is to know what you're after. If, for example, you really want to learn to defend yourself, cardio kickboxing will not get you there. You can throw all the kicks and punches you want, but air doesn't fight back. Nor will you necessarily learn the safest and most effective techniques for throwing those punches and kicks.

If you don't get your technique together, all that flailing around may feel great at the time, but may lead to long term, chronic injuries (especially in the joints) that you will never feel coming until long after they've arrived.

On the other hand, if you think real martial arts will be a good way to get a workout, well, maybe. Remember, form and technique take precedence to heavy breathing and sweat, so the intensity of the workout can vary greatly.

And (and this "And" is very important), in a dedicated martial arts facility you're going to get hit, you're going to be thrown, you may get locked down, slammed to the floor or flipped hard onto your back. Repeatedly!

Unfortunately, you can't really learn a martial arts technique until you know how it feels. And most people don't want to know.

Contrasts between dedicated facilities and fitness centers will be found in most kinds of classes. If you're more into your workout, stick with a fitness center. Just get your form together.

If you really want to learn a skill, find yourself a dedicated facility. Watch a class or two. Speak with the teacher. See if it's the right place for you.

The exception to these differences are mind—body classes. They tend to straddle the border between fitness centers and dedicated facilities.

In these classes, such as yoga and mat Pilates, equal emphasis is given both to the technique and the workout (or it should be). Since the exercise forms were created to awaken the body, strengthen and improve stability and alignment, it would seem silly to do otherwise.

The generally slower motions of many of the movements help greatly in this, as it allows the instructor more time to clearly define the technique and observe and correct the students.

Furthermore, several of these forms pursue a coming together of thought, movement and spirit, incorporating deep, rhythmic breathing, and releasing tension as the exercises are performed. (The better you focus in this manner, the sooner the body responds.)

Unless you wish to pursue such forms professionally, or in a more defined spiritual framework, these classes, taken regularly in a fitness center from the right teacher, can bring a student to a level of skill that rivals a similar student in a dedicated facility.

8. The last reason for the way classes are taught is founded on the KISS principle. To my knowledge,
    classes of this nature are native only to commercial fitness centers.

    Fitness centers like classes that can appeal to a wide range of people. They want formats that
    anyone can try, without the intimidation of learning something difficult. Straightforward, large
    muscle-based exercises that are simple to perform fit this bill beautifully.

    When the intention is to push as hard as you can, to flirt with the edge of endurance, and you're
    working with people of vastly different (or purely beginning) skills, the safest approach is to
    stick with the big motor movements of the body, using the big muscle groups in their primary
    functions. In other words, "Keep It Simple, Stupid." (No offence, that's just the acronym.)

    Classes such as spinning, calisthenics or dumbbell-based classes of various names, boot camp
    routines and others, were designed with this principle in mind. They will burn you in a hurry
    without too much worry. And they can be an exhausting lot of fun.

    Yes, there is technique to learn, and the sooner the better, but the movements are straightforward
    and the skills relatively easy to acquire. Ignore technique, however, and you'll learn firsthand
    that injuries from simple movements can be just as painful and debilitating as injuries acquired
    through more refined skills.

    How you build your body will determine what kind of body you build. If you want a sport's
    car—fast reaction, speed, dexterity, precision—you'll most likely find movement-based skills a
    helpful path. If you want a Mack truck—raw muscle, size and power—you'll probably lean toward
    bodybuilding. If a metaphysical meld of mind and muscle is your mantra, or a sinuous symbiosis
    of body and breathing, I refer you to tai chi, yoga and their various cousins.

    Still, within such general frameworks, there are innumerable ways to go. A ballerina and a
    gymnast, though pursuing similar goals, will still show many differences, not only in how the
    body is built, but also in how it moves and is supported. In bodybuilding, the specific angles of
    the working parts will directly impact how the working muscles are defined. The different forms
    within yoga and tai chi are already vast, even more so than the differences between the two
    disciplines themselves.

    Know what you're doing and why. Take it one step at a time. Form, baby, Form.

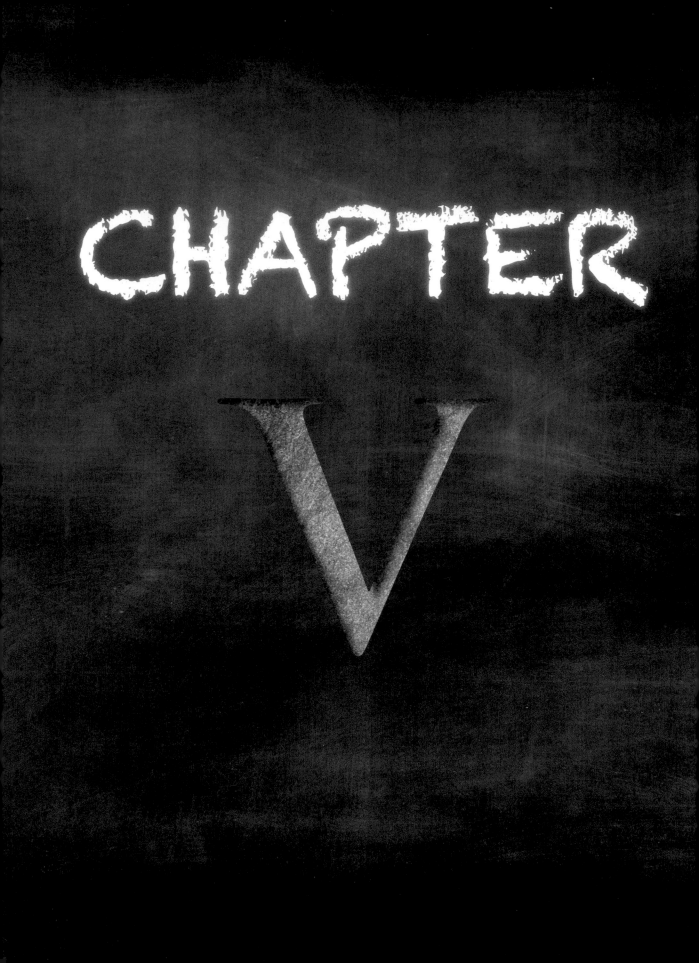

CHAPTER

V

CHAPTER V: RUNNING

Before we move on to exercises for specific parts of the body, let's take an in-depth look at one whole-body movement: running. It will provide insight into how the dynamics of movement affect the angle of the body's architecture (alignment) and support, as well as offer a good review of the mechanics of movement and breathing.

It will also prepare us for how intently we must look at each individual part of the body, in order to get the most (and safest) out of each exercise. Remember:

> "No (Motion) is an Island, entire unto Itself.
> Each is a Piece of the Main,
> a Part of the Whole"*

* An aberration of John Donne's "For Whom the Bell Tolls."
Sorry, Mr. Donne

The movement is created, controlled and sustained by numerous muscle groups. Some work together for stability. Some work in opposition, firing piston-like to maintain momentum. Still others act as heavy springs, safely absorbing the shock of the impact as the feet hit the ground.

Arms add momentum and stability by rotating forward and back in a similar—but not quite the same—manner. Working in opposition to the legs, they surge and draw from the shoulders and elbows. (Think of the mechanical arms that turn the wheels of a train—straight forward, straight back, completely stable, close to the wheels.)

The lift of the knees and the surge of the elbows are of tremendous help in moving the body. They draw the weight forward as galloping horses draw a chariot.

All these rotating parts not only must aid in support and stability, but also must maintain and control the complex movement as well. Legs and arms are primary. They can make or break your speed, comfort, safety and efficiency.

Let's start at the bottom and work our way up, examining the mechanics one section at a time.

1. First off, heel to toe. The forward leg lands on the heel, then rolls through the whole foot to push off the ball, once the body has passed.

    There may be times, however—stopping suddenly or running down a steep decline—when you find you must come down on the ball of the foot first. If that occurs, make sure you work through the heel, bringing it all the way to the ground before you push off the ball again to diminish the risk of injury.

    Think about those feet. Don't just let them flop around. They are very complex little (a relative term) machines themselves and are deserving of your close attention. Feel the weight transfer through the foot as it moves along the ground. Feel those toes as you push off the ball. Keep those feet pointed straight forward in line with the knees and in line with the run. Feet have been flying under the radar and getting off easy long enough. Time they toe the line.

2. Ankles are often a runner's weakest link. If they're not strong and aware, it only takes a sudden rise or drop in the terrain, a misstep off a curb, or the wrong pebble at the wrong time and kablooey—you're on the ground baying like a hound.

    And stability's not all you've got to worry about. The ankle is expressly responsible for controlling and guiding the foot—always in line with the knee and hip—as it works from the heel solidly through, to, and pushing off, the ball. If the ankles are not aware, strong, fluid and pliable—if they're not in control—Lookout, Moon Pie!

3. The knees and hips have it a bit easier. They have much larger muscles on stabilizer duty and somewhat less intricate roles to play in the movement. Moreover, as long as good form and technique are present, they rarely take the first hit in a destabilizing running situation.

    Along with alignment, the knees and hips play another role, indispensable to having a funky-funky good run. They are the major shock absorbers for the body. Every time a foot hits the ground, there is momentous downward gravitational force to be smoothly and evenly absorbed, as the weight passes from heel to toe, before it can again be propelled forward and out.

    The greatest load hits upon impact. The hips and knees must allow for immediate absorption (elastic control) of downward force at this time. A healthy degree of pliant resistance must be maintained in order to spring forward smoothly once the pressure is absorbed and overcome.

    A good way to understand this is to watch traffic. Study how the shock absorbers on various automobiles react. Watch how smoothly the bodies of some cars move in contrast to the wheels. Think about it when you're driving—or running—on a bumpy road.

    Build your internal shocks well!

4. Moving on to the torso: If that lower belly isn't pressing in for support, you can say goodbye to your lower back. Absorb all the shock you want in your hips, knees, and ankles, your spine is still going to share the impact of every step. Your lower spine is naturally built to take some of that impact, but when its overarched and overloaded because you aren't supporting with your lower belly that 'naturally' begets an 'un'.

    Eventually, if you don't use your lower abs, some of those softer, pretty little discs between the vertebrae of your spine are going to get squished. And, as many of us already know, squished disc means serious ouch.

    Of course, the lower belly supports the lower back much better when the upper abs are doing their job—lifting into and expanding the ribcage. This stretches the lower belly vertically as it presses in toward the lower spine, firming its elasticity in both directions. A much greater sense of stability and control is realized.

    I'm not talking about using your insides as a vacuum cleaner and sucking the upper abs in like a yogi—that training has a different purpose altogether. I'm talking about the way we did it in chapter II when working on posture. Take a deep, lifting inhale that broadens the chest and upper back; then maintain that lift and breadth with a firm, continually inward press while exhaling.

    Of course, all this ab stuff can only be done in complete cooperation with the back doing its right thing—remaining long, strong and lifted through the top of the head. This partnership of lifted abs and a lengthened spine will keep the torso controlled yet fluid—held in place, of course, with the help of strong, squared shoulders pressing down.

Often when running, there is what appears to be some mild swaying in the shoulders, in complimentary opposition to the hips. This seems natural, occuring from a slight twisting of the torso from the waist, the shoulders merely being the widest (hopefully), and therefore most obvious, visual cue. The shoulders themselves always remain squared, neither forward nor back, stabilizing the torso from the top down.

5. The arms are living pendulums anchored from the shoulders, swinging smoothly and rhythmically in opposition to the legs. The elbows move fluidly, and the forearms angling forward and slightly in toward the center line ahead of the body, through hands that are engaged yet relaxed (most folks seem to go with curled fingers or a mild fist). The palms of the hands should face each other (turning them down and back rotates the shoulders forward in caveman fashion—not good).

    If the height of the hands drops below the height of the elbows, not only is more strength required to support the forearms and hands, but, as the elbows and forearms are no longer tracking through the same space, more body surface is exposed to wind resistance. Both of these things make your run a bit harder.

    Remember, when running, the idea is to go forward. Stay streamlined. Keep your feet and knees moving front to back, don't let them—or your elbows—fly wide. Avoid swaying your body or arms from side to side. Nonlinear motion wastes strength and energy and inhibits ability.

    Everything aims forward, toward that center point just ahead of your body, splitting the air. Think motorcycle. Think bobsled. Think bullet. Stream that line.

    The level of energy required to run rises or falls in direct proportion to the efficiency of the movement. The energy available is directly related to the ability of the body's internal bellows (the lungs) to pump oxygen in and carbon dioxide out (that is to say, breathing).

6. Believe it or not, breathing requires your cooperation. Yes, it occurs without thought—involuntarily—but how well it works depends on you.

    You see, your lungs are in prison. They are serving a life sentence behind bones. The size of their cell depends on how well you lift and support through your ribcage. If you want your lungs to thrive in captivity, you've got to give them room to breathe.

    Should the myriad benefits of healthful alignment and support found in running—to joints, muscles, nerves and bones—not provide reason enough for you to do the work that cleans up your form, then do it for your lungs. Anything less than a broad, lifted open ribcage will confine your lungs to an unfulfilling life at heavy labor.

    Think about it. You've got two inflatable bags, bladders, balloons—take your pick—inside an enclosed space of changeable size. If the space contracts, inflation is limited. If the space expands, there's room to breathe more freely.

So run tall. Run expansively. No rounded shoulders, collapsed chest, tucked hips, butt backs, slack bellies, legs that never stretch or reach—these things will only add misery to the joy (and punishment) of running hard.

And don't ignore your windpipe! It matters, too. Lift tall through the back of your neck, keeping that pipe wide open. You can't fill your lungs if you can't get wind through the pipe.

It has been said that most of us use only one-third of our lungs' true potential. This suggests the lungs have a much greater capacity than many of us realize. From my own study, I can assure you that the depth—and length—of a breath can be greatly increased with practice. This comes in very handy in both high-end aerobic exertion and lengthy, slow motion moves, such as yoga. (More on breathing can be found in chapter IX, **Injury and Recovery**).

ON THE TREADMILL

Of course, many of the dangers inherent to running can be mitigated by relying on that modern mechanical beast—the treadmill. Some swear by it, some swear at it.

As for the benefits and deficits of running on a treadmill versus real-world surfaces, let us consider:

1. Treadmills are easier on your joints. They cushion your impact. They also assist your stride with their moving surfaces.

2. Treadmills have handrails for safety, minimizing the risk of slip and fall.

3. Treadmills keep you out of the icky, icky weather. (In all fairness, unless you've got a hot shower waiting, running in the pouring rain isn't that much fun. Also, running in temperatures below 26°F [-3°C] is tough on the lungs.)

4. On a treadmill, you remain in a controlled environment throughout—no traffic, no curbs, no uneven ground.

5. Treadmills are equipped with all kinds of fun gadgets that measure everything involved in your run (though I'm not convinced of their accuracy), and they keep you going at a steady pace.

6. Treadmills often face a TV, and their consoles provide a lovely, angled shelf upon which to rest your book or magazine should you choose to read during your routine.

On the other hand:

1. Real-world surfaces are what your joints are going to spend most of their time dealing with. Very few of them have the softness of a treadmill (and, when they do, the support may be quite uneven). Landing and pushing from a hard surface is a more demanding and less forgiving task. It might be helpful to get used to it.

2. As for the handrails, one is very tempted to hold onto them. Not only does this diminish the work for the arms—they no longer swing—but the entire upper body is relieved of duty and tempted to bend from the waist, dropping both shoulders and belly, not to mention both head and neck, forward. (Though sad but true, this is also seen climbing stairs). Unless you're a bellhop, or a pushcart vendor, holding the arms in this position is not something I'd recommend getting accustomed to.

3. Running in weather can be a blast. Cold and windy, hot and still, a little rain from time to time— weather lets you know you're alive. Pre-dawn, mid-afternoon, in the still of the night—keep your eyes open! Variety is a lovely thing.
    And the view! From gritty and urban to blue skies and green. You can experience some interesting, beautiful sights running outside. Build some visual memories, earn some tough weather bragging rights.

4. Yes, the environment is controlled on a treadmill. One need not be concerned with traffic, pedestrians or dangerous animals (human or otherwise). You don't need to keep your eyes open. There are no potholes, no uneven surfaces, no varied textures—gravel, mud, grass—to surprise your footing. Nothing to challenge the stability of your structure. None of those things we all encounter every day in our daily lives.

5. I've got to admit, though, those gadgets can be pretty neat. How necessary they are, I think, must be viewed case by case. Many people use the ongoing charts, graphs, measurements and such to reassure themselves that they are achieving something.
    As for keeping one running at a steady pace—or even pushing them a little—sure, treadmills can do that. However, as a trainer, I'd rather see that intention of steady-paced pushing coming solely from a deeply determined client than being helped along by a less invested machine.

6. TV is cool. Books and magazines are great. They provide great distraction. Beats the hell out of concentrating on the run, continually reviewing and improving your support, alignment, breathing and stride. I mean, who wants to be bothered with all that?

    A corporate professional I know once was telling me his new exercise plan. "I'm going to join the gym next to my office and workout during my lunch hour."

    As words of encouragement began to rise in my throat, he added, "I can make all my business calls while I exercise."

    My mouth closed of its own accord...I stood dumbfounded.

    As an afterthought, he added, "It doesn't really make a difference whether or not you concentrate on your exercise, does it?"

    I couldn't believe an intelligent, educated, full-grown adult would even consider such a question. I asked him what would happen if he didn't concentrate on his business, and he seemed surprised I thought that a legitimate comparison.

Well that's it. More than you ever wanted to think about running. Thing is, if you're going to run, the only way to achieve a reliable, safe form is to examine and train the individual parts until you've got them doing what you want. Which is to say, working together in happy harmony.

Now, let's get down to specific parts of the body.

CHAPTER

VI

CHAPTER VI: EXERCISES

HIPS, LEGS AND FEET

I write this title from the hips down to indicate the direction of thinking necessary when governing the lower body. One may follow one's vagabond feet wherever they wish to go, but those feet should be vagabound from the hips down.

Assuming that the hips are properly aligned below the torso, their positioning of the knees—with the feet following, of course—have a direct and lasting impact on the abilities, health and lifespan of the joints and muscles involved. Get the architecture wrong and not only will your lower limbs suffer. Once in pain, the compensations you make below will also distort everything above.

It takes training, but mostly in the way one thinks. The muscular and structural issues for most people's hips, knees and feet tend to be pretty basic. Often, a small realignment makes all the difference.

Just a few months' concentration on a 24/7 basis and your muscles will begin to regularly remember what you want them to do. The only real difficulty is in getting your mind to keep it in mind 24/7 until it sticks.

The hips determine not only the direction of the knees (and therefore feet), but also the width and distance between the legs. Equally essential is the hips' role in stabilizing the legs as they support or move weight.

How they are used as stabilizers directly impacts the distribution of the weight

- on the muscles of the legs (front of the thigh versus back, front of the calves versus back, inside versus outside, upper end versus lower end, front of the calves versus back, deep muscle versus surface),
- on the knees (degree of stress in the joint; stability and alignment),
- on the ankles (stress, stability and alignment) and
- on the feet (left foot/right foot, heels to toes, inside of the feet/outside of the feet).

Stability in the hips is accomplished through the cooperation of various muscles in the butt, the upper, outer and inner thighs and the lower belly, back and waist.

With the exception of the lower belly, when the lower body is worked, these other muscles tend to activate, at least to some extent, regardless of conditioning. That lower belly, though, if you aren't consciously training it, will just sag, bag and generally ruin your day.

We'll get to more about the belly in the next section, but, for now, if your lower body is working and your belly isn't helping your hips, your hips won't be doing right by your lower body. A slack lower belly inhibits the full and appropriate engagement of the inner thighs and the outside corners of the lower butt, and these failings will cause endless problems in your future.

BUTTS, BUTTS, BUTTS

Due to the overwhelming interest—throughout human history, it seems—in this particular feature of our anatomy, I feel, before we look at exercises, a special word must be given to these rumptious rounds of misery and delight.

So many people worry about their own (or someone else's), obsess over their own (or someone else's), wonder why their (or someone else's) doesn't do what they want it to or look how they want it to.

Thing is, regarding your own, if you treat it right, it will do its best for you. (The someone else's will have to take care of its own.) Just remember, how you work it has a huge impact on the shape it assumes.

THE DIRECTION OF THE KNEES

If you want more of that round, apple-cheeked look, keep your knees and toes forward when you work. Do lots of squats and lunges. If reducing size isn't an issue, add some resistance. Work through those heels!

If you'd like more lift from the bottom and more contoured sides, try squats with the knees and toes rotated open from the hips (yeah, like pliés in ballet). As you squat, make sure the butt stays vertically above the heels. To rise, press the heels toward the ground. If the butt remains vertically above the heels, the body will be forced upward.

Concentrate on squeezing the butt in from the sides as you rise. Once the knees are straight, rise onto your toes, keeping the open rotation in the knees and feet. At the top, stretch long through the top of the head and squeeze the—mild expletive here—out of your butt and lower belly.

To work harder, draw the heels closer together. Keep your butt directly above your heels and the weight securely on the balls of the feet at all times. This requires practice.

For the uninitiated, the lower one goes in this position, the harder it is to maintain proper form. The knees begin to roll in or wobble, the butt wants to push back, stability is compromised as the joints move out of line—very stressful.

Keep your whole body vertically aligned and strongly supported at all times. And, if you want to keep your knees healthy, work through those heels.

Now, let's take some basic exercises and talk alignment, support and weight distribution.

SQUATS

Although the width between the legs varies depending on the goal, most people have the easiest time with squats when their legs are approximately one-and-a-half times as wide as their hips. Any wider than two times this, can be dangerous to the knees when bending them. (A narrower stance raises similar stability and weight distribution issues.)

At one-and-a-half times the width, the challenges are clear, but not overwhelming. It's easier to feel what needs to be done:

1. Stand tall, knees straight. Support with the butt by lightly squeezing, with the lower abs pressing in and the upper abs lifting (Photo 30). Your shoulders press down to secure the lift of the torso—aligned vertically over the sides of the hips, neither pulled back nor rolled forward. Your head lifts long through the crown and the muscles on the back of the neck. For now, put your hands on your hips.

2. Your legs will get their best work if the feet are pointed straight ahead.

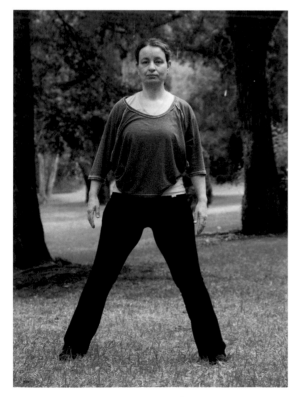

This makes the muscles work their hardest and lets you really feel how the hips and inner thighs govern alignment as the knees bend.

Turning the feet slightly open will make squats easier both in strength and in aligning the knees. If you need to turn the feet out a bit at first, that's okay. However, do not turn them out beyond the knees' ability to line up above them.

PHOTO 30

3. Keeping the torso tall and lifted, bend your knees. Reach forward with the arms to counterbalance the weight shift (don't let your shoulders roll forward). This motion works the upper arms, shoulders, upper torso, and abs. (If the shoulders reach forward or lift with the arms, both of which tend to round the upper back, there is little to be gained but a reinforced bad habit.) The direction of the palms—up, down, turned in or out, will affect how the upper body is worked.

Put the weight on your heels as you go down (Photo 31). (The torso must bend forward a bit from the hips to compensate for the shift of weight to the heels. Be sure to keep your back straight and head aligned.)

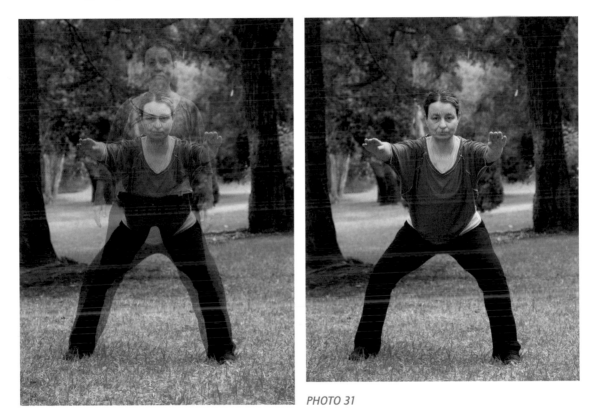

PHOTO 31

4. Keep a close eye on your knees. Press open from the inner thighs to hold them properly in line with the balls of the feet. Be sure that they never pass the front of the toes (keep your weight in your heels).

Many people—when first attempting to press their bending knees open over the balls of their feet, with the feet straight ahead as they squat—find that the support of their weight shifts to the outsides of their feet. This happens because the ankles lack the training to make the independent adjustment to the new position of the knees. It takes a few weeks for them to come around.

5. The deeper you squat, the more work required to maintain a lifted torso (one that bends forward only from the hips). There is a tendency, especially among the less flexible, for both the upper back and the shoulders to round forward in a reaching manner, relieving the lower abs and back of their responsibility.

    Also, lower abs, when left to their own devices, will slack considerably as you go down. Teach them a better way.

6. At the lowest you can go with good form (no more than a 90-degree bend in the knees), reverse direction and press up through the butt and the back of the legs. The bulk of the weight remains on the heels throughout. Pay special attention to your knees as you change direction, as they very often roll in a bit at the point of transition (the most unstable point mechanically). Don't let this happen to you.

7. Supporting through the torso, return to a vertical stance.

8. For a great variation, turn the knees and toes open as wide as the knees will allow (Photo 32). Work the hip rotators as you open and bend the knees (Photo 33). Be sure to keep the knees in line with the opened feet.

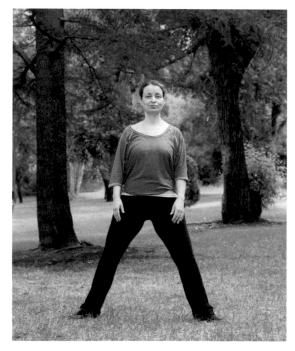
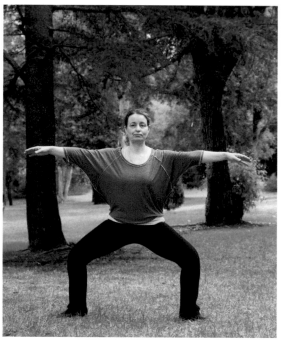

PHOTO 32   PHOTO 33

LUNGES

Though the obvious motion of a lunge is in the legs, the work is primarily in the lower abs and the hips (the core, if you like). The farther you step out (within your safe ability, of course), the more these engage and the stronger you become.

Short-step lunges, although often perceived as easier by beginners, actually put unhealthful stress in the forward knee and make stabilizing the hips and torso a much dicier proposition. Your muscles may work less, but your structure pays a heavy price. (Short-step lunges of any real depth should be left to those who have trained in the techniques to deal with them.)

When lunging, always go for the long step:

1. Stand with the feet under the hips, the body properly aligned. Hands on the waist (Photo 34).

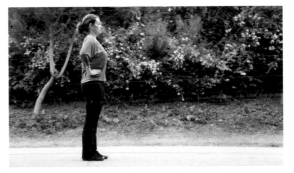

PHOTO 34

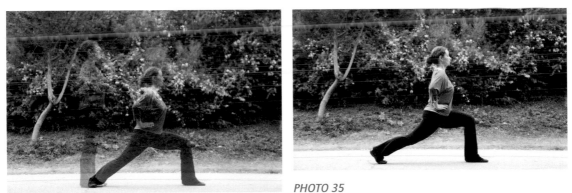

PHOTO 35

2. When stepping forward into a lunge, work from the hips and lower belly. Take a long step out, with the back heel vertically aligned with the back knee (the back knee relaxes a bit, but does not bend as you step).
   Bring the weight onto the heel of the forward foot and drop your hips (forward and down) toward that heel, with the chest lifted and the belly squeezing all the way (Photo 35).
   Do not let the knee pass the front of the toes. nor shift the weight onto the front of the front foot.

When stepping back into a lunge, work from the hips and lower belly. Keep the weight just forward of the heel of the front foot. Drop your hips vertically and reach back with the moving leg. Don't let your forward knee move out beyond the toes or back behind the ankle. Try to keep the front calf just forward of vertical throughout.

In both cases, squeeze that lower belly throughout the move. Keep your upper torso strong and lifted—stretching the spine—all the way through the top of the head. Keep your shoulders securely in place.

3.   Be sure that the back knee and foot are in alignment with each other. The back knee should face the ground. The raised back heel should be vertically aligned above the ball of the foot (although either may be a bit forward, depending on the reach and depth of the lunge).

At the full range of the lunge, the back knee can be stretched by pressing the back heel backward as the hips press forward and down toward the front heel. If the lower abs are not strongly engaged in this, however, the lower back will suffer.

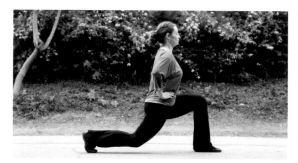

PHOTO 36

The back knee may also be bent once at full range, bringing it down to, or as close to, the ground as safely as possible (Photo 36). Bending the back knee, then stretching it again as you rise, challenges you in a different way.

The greatest challenge when bending the back knee comes in keeping the heel and knee working together. The knee must continually face the ground and maintain a straight line of support from the hip through the (vertically) raised heel, with the weight on the ball of the foot.

It is very common to feel that your back knee and heel are vertically aligned when, actually, they are turned open somewhat. The heel tends to open the most, and the knee, which almost always remains bent to some degree, hangs lost somewhere between the line of the hip and the heel. This is extremely dangerous for the lower inside corner of the knee—the spot that usually takes the greatest stress in this aberration of form—and promotes a lazy and unhelpful memory for the muscles of the ankles.

The back heel requires special attention. For many reasons—it's stretched out behind you, it's out of your field of vision, it's the farthest thing away from your core and supports far less weight than the forward foot—it's the last thing you think of.

Bent knee or not, once vertically aligned, that troublesome back ankle may want to roll open and take the weight to the outside of the foot. It takes a lot of practice to get and stay on the ball of the foot, but that practice will help insure the strength and safety of your ankles and knees for years to come.

4. When rising to the front foot, everything stays solidly engaged, with full support from the butt and belly, while the weight is pressed forward and up through the heel of the front foot (with some initial assistance from the back leg and foot), much in the way one climbs a stair or rises from a squat.

When rising to the back foot, there is some initial push from the ball of the front foot before the back leg takes over. Be careful not to stress the front knee joint as you do this. Squeeze your butt and belly to draw the leg in.

If you are performing walking lunges—moving forward with each new step—you will find it much easier to stabilize if you bring your feet together and pause each time before stepping out again.

There is another way of lunging that few people use (outside of some classes), which has particular benefits of its own. Unless you're into yoga, ballet, or certain fighting techniques, you may not be have tried it out.

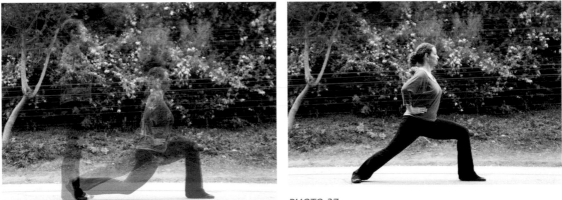

PHOTO 37

In this lunge, the back foot turns open, up to 90 degrees, and the back leg remains rigidly straight as you lunge forward (Photo 37).

This is the standard version. For a combat exercise, initially bend the back leg, with the feet slightly wider than hip-width, then stretch it with speed and force, pushing hard from the back foot to ballistically thrust the body forward. The back foot must remain flat on the ground throughout the exercise. It should never be rolled onto its inside edge.

If this is done—or if the foot is opened beyond 90 degrees—considerable instability is introduced to the inside of the back leg, the very part of the leg that is already working the hardest. Both pinpoint injuries to and over-stretching of the joints become readily available if one is not very careful.

This type of lunge for the back leg focuses the work in the inner thigh—both in strength and flexibility—as well as challenges strength and control to achieve and maintain a thoroughly straight back knee. If that back knee bends or that back heel rises, or if the back foot rolls onto its inside edge, watch out! Keep that knee straight, keep that foot flat! It must be solidly anchored to the ground.

A special note here on the mechanics of rotating the back knee when lunging, whether it is locked straight and open, or facing the ground with a vertically raised back heel: It's all in the hips.

The hips are diagonal to the front when the foot and knee are open. Rotate the hips straight ahead, and the foot and heel are inclined to rotate vertically. The hips control the movement.

As with squats, adding upper-body work to lunges brings a whole new appreciation to the move. Just be sure your lunging form is ready for the additional challenge.

If you really get your lunges and squats together, they will give you a good foundation from which to approach any lower-body moves.

KNEES, SPECIFICALLY

My personal belief is that the knees get their best work when being used in whole- and lower-body movements. That's what's natural. That's where technique needs to be perfect; that's what gets you through life. Practical applications.

Having said that, there is, most definitely, a place for isolated knee exercise. Such a specific focus can be helpful in all aspects of the joint's integrity.

There is one particular movement, Calf Extensions, that, when done properly, helps correctly align the joint, while strengthening and tightening the muscles that wrap around it (to hold the structural alignment in place).

CALF EXTENSIONS

1. Sit in a chair with good lower back and thigh support. The chair should be at a height that places your thighs parallel to the floor (Photo 38).

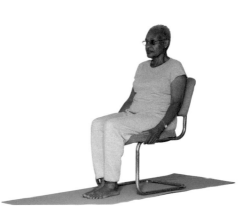

PHOTO 38

2. Sit tall and don't let your belly sag. Hold the sides of the chair, if you wish, to add stability. Slowly extend one leg out straight, squeeze lightly, then lower (Photo 39).

3. Try the other leg.

4. Keep it up, at least 10 reps each leg.

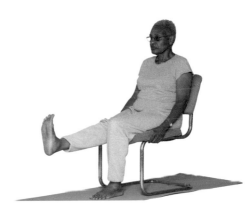

PHOTO 39

5. If it doesn't bother your lower back, try both legs together (Photo 40).
   Work the toes as well.

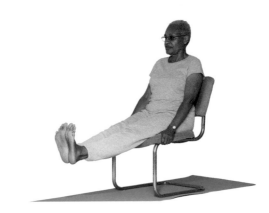

PHOTO 40

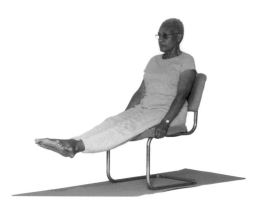

PHOTO 41

How about pointing (Photo 41)?

6. Try rotating the knee open (heels together) from the hips with the legs stretched.

There is a standard machine at virtually every exercise facility, which performs this same function and allows extra resistance to be added to the move, which can be a good thing. Just don't get carried away.

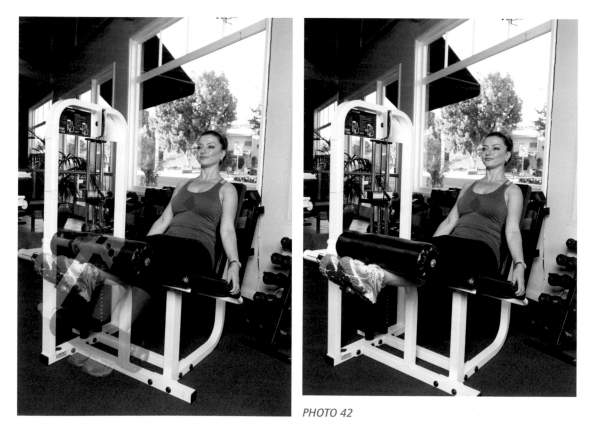

PHOTO 42

When using added resistance of any kind, the knees must remain aligned in the direction of the work, in this case, vertical (Photo 42).

Some people perform this exercise with ankle weights attached. That's fine, so long as the weights aren't very heavy and the feet are flat on the ground when the muscles around the knee are disengaged. The knee isn't really built to have extra weight hanging down from it—pulling it apart, as it were (just ask anyone who's been drawn and quartered). The knees are built to withstand compression.

However this exercise is performed, the legs should remain within the breadth of the hips.

An easier variation is to do this exercise lying flat on your back.

1. Knees bend vertically, feet on the floor (Photo 43).

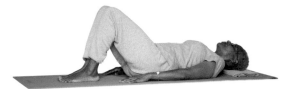

PHOTO 43

2. Extend the leg—or legs—skyward (Photo 44).

3. Stretch those knees. Use your feet. Do your reps.

PHOTO 44

Just remember to extend the leg all the way to get the full benefits of knee extensions as a part of your complete and hearty breakfast. Mmmmm—knee extensions!

"Eine letzte Nachricht", as the Germans say—one last note. Many instructors, when teaching knee extensions, include holding the knee(s) at full extension for what amounts to a few seconds (deep breath, count to five, etc.).

If you're lying flat on the floor and your legs are vertically aligned above the hips, no prob. But if you're seated or on a diagonal, depending on conditioning or genetics, holding that stretched position for any amount of time—or even lifting both legs simultaneously—can cause lower, or sometimes middle, back pain. Not a good thing.

You got to know when to hold 'em and know when to fold 'em.

CALVES AND ANKLES AND FEET (OH MY)

There is a standard leg machine for strengthening the calves that offers a great chance to strengthen the alignment of the ankles and feet as well. Curiously enough, it's called the Calf Raise Machine.

CALF RAISE MACHINE

Sit, legs forward, knees bent at 90 degrees. Vertical resistance (weight) is applied to the top of the thighs (Photo 45). Then press the heels up, lifting the weight (Photo 46).

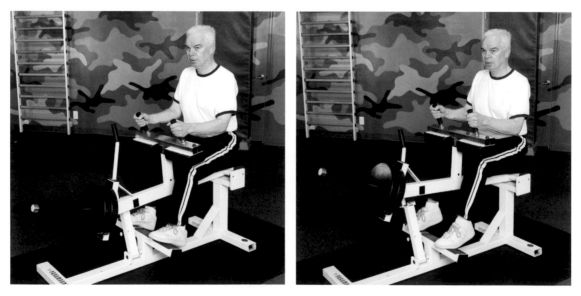

PHOTO 45   *PHOTO 46*

A joyous little squeeze in the calves at the top of the move and you're back down to try it again.

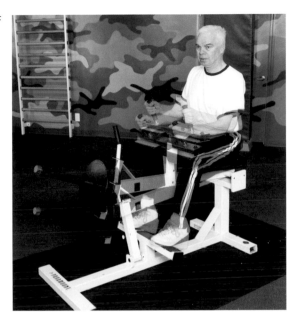

This simple machine, though primarily used for strength and size gains in the large muscle at the back of the calves, is excellent for practicing the correct alignment of the ankles and feet. Just concentrate on pressing up through the balls of the feet and overcome the inclination (literally and figuratively) of the ankles to roll to the outside—or, in rare cases, to the inside—of the foot.

The secure pressure of the weight on the tops of the thighs—it only moves up and down—is very stabilizing to the pressing calves, ankles and feet, allowing one to really feel the work and to consider the alignment of the load to make corrections as necessary.

It's a great way to recognize, and equalize, the workings of the inner and outer stabilizers in these lower portions of your lower limbs.

This area of the body can be similarly worked for stability and strength—though not necessarily size—by using a step, or some other platform, a least a couple of inches higher than the ground.

STANDING CALF RAISE

1. With your feet hip-width apart, stand with toes straight ahead and with the full pads of the front of your feet firmly on the step. The heels hang off the back. The legs are strong and the knees are stretched (Photo 47).

2. Support with your arms by holding on to a bar, the back of a chair or pressing against a wall. The support should be about waist high, but, if you're using a wall, keep the hands at the approximate height of the solar plexus. For greatest stability, the hands should be a bit wider than the shoulders. Be sure the rest of your body is nice and tall, strong and lifted, doing the right thing.

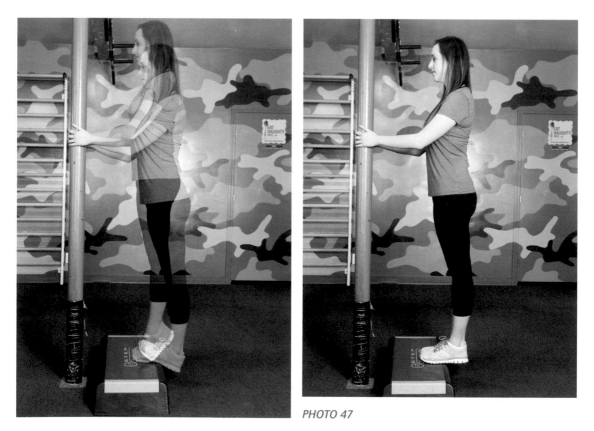

PHOTO 47

3. Squeeze your butt, your belly and your thighs and stretch your knees, pressing strongly into the balls of your feet and rising (forward and up) onto your toes.

4. Really stretch the legs. Work from the lower belly and hips, down through those strong, stretched knees. (The ankles and feet can't do their job without solid support from above.)

5. Now use the insides and outsides of the calves to stabilize those ankles in vertical perfection over the balls of the feet (Photo 48).

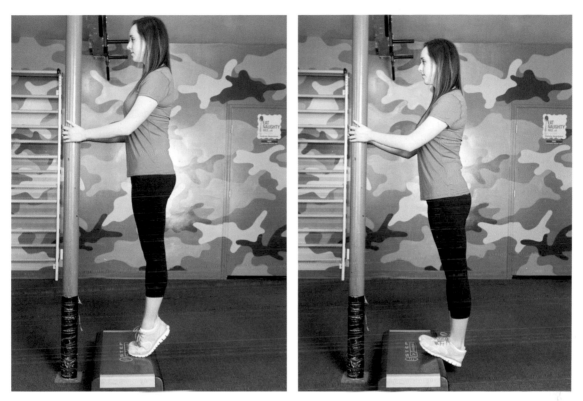

PHOTO 48   PHOTO 49

6. Once aligned, think about stretching those feet as far as they can go. (Careful, now...)

7. Still lifting—from the top of the head through every (other) part of your body—slowly, with control and strength, lower your heels. Think of stretching the heels down against the lift from the top of the head and the rest of the body.

8. To the degree that it feels safe, allow your heels to drop below the edge of the step (Photo 49). Do not relax the muscles but rather keep them engaged.

9. Repeat 10 times or more.

That ought to get you going. Just keep a few things in mind:

First, if the exercise bothers your stretched knees, you must readjust your weight or relax them a bit (let them soften). If it bothers your back, look to your abs and, possibly, your shoulders.

Second, the more (farther or harder) you stretch your ankles and feet, and the more you stretch your calves by dropping the heels, the more likely you are to get a strain, cramp or pull in one or more of the muscles and tendons involved, especially if you're not used to working them under such isolated stress.

Third, to challenge yourself further in this exercise, try some of these variations:

1. Work with the legs and feet all the way together (touching each other) rather than with the feet hip-width apart. This provides greater insight into the role of the butt, hips, lower belly and inner thighs as stabilizers, while increasing the challenge to the ankles to remain aligned.

2. Take one hand off the bar and move the other to the center of the bar (as you face it). This places the supporting hand roughly in front of the navel (or the solar plexus, if against a wall), in the middle of the body. This decreases the stability provided by the arms, while increasing your sensitivity to the (vertical) centerline of your abs, which makes them easier to feel as you work. Greater stability must then be generated through the lower abs, butt and inner and outer thighs to compensate.

3. Rather than face the bar, turn 90 degrees to the left or right. The outer hand goes to the waist, the inner to the bar. The hand on the bar should be placed palm down. The elbow should be slightly forward of the shoulder.
   If the elbow gets behind the shoulder, the shoulder will rotate forward, the torso will twist, or both, misaligning and destabilizing the body.
   Try not to grip the bar too hard as you work. Make your body stabilize properly and use the hand on the bar as a back-up for when all else fails. A light, relaxed touch on the bar will keep your shoulder and elbow relaxed and in position and keep your focus on the lifting legs and torso, instead of in a desperately gripping hand.

Isolated calf exercises are fine, if you feel you need them, and they can be very helpful. Just remember to use those calves in plenty of whole-body work as well. That's where they really shine.

WALKING AND RUNNING

If reducing your size is important, hard running or brisk walking, preferably on a flat surface, is the fastest (ahem!) way I know to achieve this. Running on a flat surface allows you to work the muscles of your backside exclusively through forward motion, without the added weight of gravity that comes when pushing uphill (see following section on stairs and hills). Running on the flat, your heart rate, heavy breathing and sweat—while you propel rather than lift your weight—can burn you and your bum down to nothing but long, lean muscle in a hurry, relatively speaking.

Keep in mind, though, the muscles of the butt also work very differently in walking and running.

When you walk, you rise up and over your forward leg, cresting as you pass your foot. When running, the opposite occurs. You bend the forward knee and press down into the ground, pushing up and out again as you pass your foot (the height of the body is at its lowest when you pass over your foot). Different muscles fire differently to achieve these different techniques.

For regular exercise, either running or brisk walking can be fine. It depends on what you want, what you are capable of, and how hard you're willing to work.

If you intend to run, though, don't spend your running time walking. Always maintain your running form. When you're out of breath, don't stop or walk, just slow down as much as you need—even down to walking speed—until you recover your breath. Just keep your running form.

STAIRS AND HILLS

If the size of your caboose is not an issue, stairs or hills can be great. Just remember two things: The angle of push determines how your muscles work, and the heavier the load, the bigger your muscles are likely to build.

Consider stair machines. I see a lot of people dragging (what seems to me) excess baggage up those stairs, and I imagine at least some of them want to reduce their payload. I'm just not convinced that climbing stairs or hills is the best way to go.

Look at the angle of the work—pushing forward and up, rising to a higher place. The resistance of gravity is added to the weight of moving the body. A mild, steady rise may not be a big deal, but get up to 20 or 25 degrees, and it soon becomes heavy work.

Although, at more severe angles, a strong, lifted forward bend from the waist may prove helpful in the climb, even at lower angles on hills and—chronically—on stairs, the body seems inclined (yes, I know...) to droop at the shoulders, stoop at the waist and let the belly sway in the breeze, hanging slackly from the gallows of the ribs' cruel cage.

All the same, your hips and thighs can become very powerful climbing stairs and hills. And you can burn a whole bunch of calories and reduce your body fat. But, reduce fat as you might, you're also building muscle. Though muscle only takes one-third the space of fat, build enough and you'll replace more than reduce.

Consider the Olympic speed skater. Consider his or her form—bent forward from the waist, pushing down and back. The technique is very similar to stair climbing. (Although moving along a flat surface, the skaters' low bend at the waist adds considerable load to the hips and thighs.)

Now, look at those (speed skating) hips and thighs. Powerful, yes—lean, yes—and massive.

Consider the general pear of their shape. It's not too different from what can come from climbing stairs. And, if that's what you want, it's a beautiful thing.

When thinking about how to work your backside, look around. What professionals—athletes, body-builders, performers—have the shape you're looking for? What do they do? What would you like?

There are so many ways to activate the backside. Learn to use it wisely. Every whole-body movement and any number of more isolated exercises require its direct participation. One area in which this is true deals with the abdominals.

THOSE CRAZY ABDOMINALS

Although the visible "abs" are actually one long, sectioned muscle (the *abdominis rectus*), as different approaches can be used to work different sections, I will stick with the common plurality.

There is also another, though less well known. The *transverse abdominis*, which lies beneath the visible one and wraps across the body, somewhat like your own personal lap band. A partially involuntary muscle, it defines the base of what the media commonly refer to as "the core".

It seems there are as many ways to work the abs—and their many loyal supporters—as there are people to work them. As always, how they are worked has a huge impact on how they are shaped.

Although ab exercises can be performed at various angles (on an incline bench, for instance) or with varying degrees of support (a strong surface supporting the hips and lower back versus no surface at all—as in hanging upside down), not everyone can do these safely. The examples given here are performed on the floor—a flat, solid surface being the safest way I know to do them.

AB WORK AND THE NECK

There is a lot of controversy surrounding the role of the head and neck when doing ab work, particularly Crunches and Sit-ups, and professionals are split in their decisions.

One school of thought goes for rolling the head up, purely from the neck's own power, with the arms folded across the curling torso. Others feel that the head should be kept "neutral" (a somewhat inaccurate term), which means that the neck doesn't intentionally bend, but rather stays as straight as possible, usually stabilized by the fingers at the back of the skull, with the elbows pressed wide.

If rolling the unsupported neck up by its own power feels good, no problem. Most people will eventually find it straining (lift your head up and down off your pillow a couple dozen times and see if it makes you happy). Your head's a heavy piece of goods. Sometimes, a little support goes a long way.

Keeping the neck neutral is often cited as a way to really isolate the abs in their work. Even if that were true, does this extra isolation make them work any harder or with increased sensitivity? Perhaps it just diminishes the natural strengthening and aligning movements of the neck, which, in normal circumstances, curls along with the spine.

Pain is another reason given for working with a neutral neck. While it is true this position can mitigate the pain of pre-existing neck injury while doing Crunches and Sit-ups, that comfort comes at a price.

If the natural movements of the neck cause soreness, it seems to me that the soreness should be understood and addressed, rather than just accepting a limited range of motion. A neutral neck isn't, to my mind, going to improve a sore neck and could conceivably make it worse, weakening the muscles of the neck and, subsequently, the alignment of the spine.

Also, when the neck is neutral, the higher the torso rises from the floor, the harder one is pressed not to let the chin jut forward. A jutting chin causes the upper spine to arch as the lower spine curls, with both under stress. Somewhere, between the two, the spine will have to resolve this schism, and the resolution may not be a fun one.

What used to be common, but seems to have fallen out of favor, was to support the head with the hands—fingers interlaced—at the back of the skull (much as one would hold a heavy bowl from underneath) and allow the neck to curl naturally with the rest of the spine.

The problem with this last one is that people are inclined to pull the body up from the arms and shoulders rather than curling from the belly. This diminishes results for the abs and stresses the boo-yah out of the muscles and bones of the neck and upper shoulders, causing all kinds of unhappiness.

It is my understanding that these first two methods of handling the neck (described previously) were conceived initially as attempts to get around this desire of the arms and shoulders to pull. If such is the case, then I believe these methods are missing the point. To me, it recalls the old, "Doc, it hurts when I do 'that'"—"Then don't do 'that' anymore" thing.

My response would be different. I would try to learn to do 'that' safely (presuming it's not an unnatural act). In this case of Sit-ups, I would try to learn with the natural movement of the body and let my neck curl forward with the rest of my spine.

I would have to quit thinking from my hands and arms and learn to curl from my belly. I would keep my shoulders strongly in place and teach my hands and arms to support rather than pull. If I could achieve those things, my neck and shoulders would be safer, smarter and capable of more adventurous challenges.

Your abs and their friends (collectively, the core) are the guys who take care not only of your spine, but support your organs as well. They need your support to give you their own.

STANDARD CRUNCH

In a lean body, a fair amount of definition can be had just by doing enough Crunches. (I differentiate Crunches from Sit-ups by the rule that, when doing Crunches, the lower back does not lift off the ground, whereas in a Sit-up, the whole body rises.)

1. Lie flat on your back, knees bent vertically to 90 degrees (Photo 50).

   The knees line up with the hips and feet, which are hip-width apart, feet flat on the ground, toes forward. (Viewed from above, you should see a straight line from the hips through the knees and ankles to the balls of the feet). The lower back is flat on the floor.

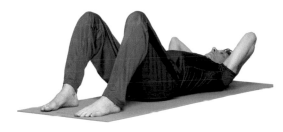

PHOTO 50

2. The hands reach behind the head and the fingers interlace to support the weight of the head and prevent stressing the neck. (See the previous section on ab work and the neck.) The elbows are forward in front of the shoulders. This diminishes the desire to whip them in, from wide open, and pull with the shoulders as the body curls up.

3. Squeeze the abs, roll the body into itself and up, from the head—don't pull with those arms—to the lower back, which remains on the floor (Photo 51).

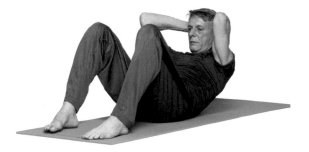

PHOTO 51

Rather than thinking "up," think of curling your upper body toward your hips. It's a truer description of what the abs are actually doing and will give you a better focus. The "up" is, basically, a by-product of the angle.

As you curl, feel the work roll through your abs from the top down. Do your best to press the abs in and not out.

As you roll up, there will be some forward motion of the elbows and shoulders. As long as you're not pulling, but merely supporting the head, this is fine. The body is simply shifting weight into the direction of the move to minimize undue stress.

4. At the top, reverse your direction and roll the back down to the floor. Keep the vertebrae of the spine descending in consecutive order. The back of the head (back of the hands) is the last thing to reach the ground.

5. Repeat as often as necessary.

Crunch though you might, what can be gained by Crunches alone is somewhat limited. Since the hips and legs are not active in the movement (they remain stationary throughout), the lower abs are not fully activated. This means Crunches are not likely to flatten your belly below the navel. It will be more inclined to pooch out a bit. Maintaining proper support in daily life will require more attention.

SIT-UPS

Rising all the way up onto the butt—Sit-ups—can help with that, depending on your form. The position of the knees and feet in relation to the hips and belly are crucial as to whether the lower belly works hard and wants to press out or in as it works.

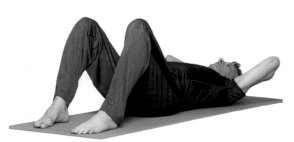

1. The starting position is the same as for Crunches (steps 1 and 2) (Photo 52). Doing Sit-ups with the legs out straight is ill advised, as the lower back is arched in this position and needs to curl in the move.

PHOTO 52

2. Squeeze those abs and rise, constantly curling toward the hips. As the lower back lifts, think chest to the knees.

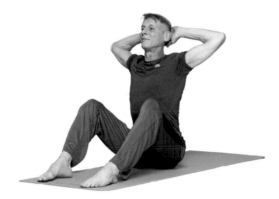

PHOTO 53

Try to avoid using the tops of the thighs to do the work. If you can, at the top, give an extra lift forward and up, from the lower back through the top of the head, as you broaden the chest and press the elbows wide (Photo 53).

Try to achieve, for one brief moment, a completely straight—though not necessarily vertical—lower-back (the knees may press wide a touch at this juncture).

Flexibility and muscular ability may be issues At the very least, avoid jutting your chin forward at the top of each rep. Challenges, challenges.

Most people will require some assistance or resistance applied to the feet—at the ankles—to be able to raise the torso past a crunch. One person does Sit-ups while another holds their feet down, or one's feet may be placed under an appropriately heavy, stable and supportive resistance.

Be careful that the resistance presses from the top of the foot—where it joins the leg—diagonally down towards the heel. If the pressure on the top of the foot is forward of this point, an overstressing of the top of the foot can occur, which will leave you with some very interesting burning pain, soreness and (possible) weakness in the area.

The extent to which one can sit up, and the extent to which one can keep the knees in line with the hips and feet, is affected by flexibility, but even more so by the girth of one's belly. A big belly gets in the way of the rest of the body rising up and forces the knees wide as one rises.

This is unfortunate for three reasons. First, opening the knees diminishes support—from the legs and hips—to the rising body. At the same time, opening the knees takes the work out of the center of the belly (which, in such cases, needs the most work) and puts it in the sides, hips and back. Finally, opening the knees takes alignment work away from the inner thighs—another area often weaker than it should be.

Why not just open the feet wider, you might ask, and keep an angled line of support from the hips down? Sure, but feet wider than your hips cause the belly to work less and less higher you go.

In Sit-ups, the torso's muscles tend to work in the line of the legs. Feet and knees all the way together—the middle line of the belly cranks throughout. Hip-width apart, full on abs from top to bottom. Feet wider than the hips—it starts with the upper abs, then moves the workload into the sides and back the higher you rise. The poor little (a speculative term) lower belly is relegated to marginal involvement.

Remember, whatever you do—throughout all of this—your hands support your head to protect the neck. They (and the shoulders) **never** pull on it to get your body up. Our bodies are drawn to enough bad habits without encouraging more.

3. One has to be careful coming down from a full Sit-up. There is a strong urge to let the lower back drop rapidly to the ground, and neither the implicit lack of control in this, nor the impact of each thud, is good for you.
    Very often, the hardest part of the exercise is not when the muscles are squeezing together, but when they are controlling the release. You've got to really work to control the descent of the lower back. Once it is down, the release from the rest of the curl comes more easily.
    (P.S. The majority of people I've witnessed crunching and sitting-up never bring their heads [the back of their hands] all the way to the ground. Some get close, but most don't even do that. Bringing the head down—all the way—provides an extra little bit of resisted stretch to the abs—especially the upper abs, right down through the center of the body. Such little touches make a big difference.)

For all the benefits of **Sit-ups** to the abs, once the lower back is off the floor, natural body mechanics cause a majority of the workload to be taken over by the lower back and hip flexors. That's fine—it's good, healthy work, and strengthening those muscle groups is necessary to any sincere soul seeking true ab-solution. But, at that point, the abs are no longer the body's primary mover. It's up to you to make them squeeze their hardest.

Keep in mind, though, Sit-ups can be very stressful on the lower back. **Crunches**, on the other hand, done properly, are very safe. Yet **Crunches** don't help that lower belly so much.

Maybe it's time we tried some **Leg Lifts**.

Leg Lifts are one of the most misunderstood exercises out there. "I can't do those, they hurt my lower back" is a cry that can be heard throughout the land. Thing is, leg lifts can be excellent for the lower back—and, of course, the lower belly—but only if they're done right.

Flexibility is often an issue, but, for most, it can be improved while doing the work. Same with strength—there are varying degrees of difficulty, so one can start off easy. The big players in **Leg Lifts**, the ultimate makers of safety or breakers of backs, are architecture and support: how you build the **Leg Lifts**; how much you stress your lower back; and how you use the angle of the legs bending at the hips to control, strengthen, and improve your base (the lower back stabilized by the lower belly) instead of injuring it.

Many people begin their Leg Lifts lying more or less flat on the ground, legs extended though not particularly engaged (not strong and stretched from the butt and belly down through the foot). Some, thinking to maintain the arch of the lower back, put their hands under their lower backs to support it.

From this casual, supine posture, they dead lift the (now at least partially engaged—it's automatic) legs, forcing an arched lower spine to curl against itself into the very center of the pressure of all that lifting weight. To make things worse, the extended legs put the moving weight all the way out on the feet, as far from the hips as can be—forcing a very heavy dead lift indeed.

Can you hear those spinal discs crunch, Cap'n? Sound like a good idea to you?

Perhaps try a Leg Lift—that's a little less stressful.

SINGLE-LEG LIFTS

1. The beginning posture is the same as for Crunches and Sit-ups (step 1), except that the arms are placed by the sides of the body.

2. The shoulders press down into the body (not the floor—this arches the chest). The forearms press flat against the ground—palms down—near the hips (Photo 54). For more support, wedge the hands (palms down) under the bottom of the butt, where it leaves the floor at the top of the legs. Do not put your hands under your lower back!.

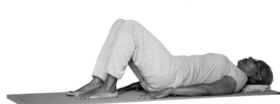

PHOTO 54

3. Press the lower back flat into the floor. Stretch the spine comfortably, long through the top of the head.

4. To begin, press the lower belly and the lower back into the ground and curl your rising knee up and in, over your belly, to just beyond your navel (toward the chest) (Photo 55).
    The weight of the working leg should now be resting comfortably over your body's center of gravity.

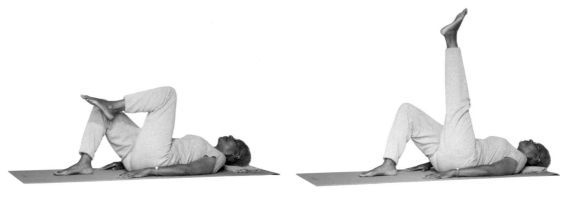

PHOTO 55   PHOTO 56

5. With the knee as far up as it is willing to go—over a flat, stable lower back—extend the lower leg upward (stretch from the knee), and try to straighten the leg completely (Photo 56).

    Either point or flex the foot (your hips, back and belly will achieve much more specificity and definition—and more safely—if you do). Remember, true stability requires all the working bits to be thoughtfully engaged.

6. Lower your leg at a smooth and even pace, descending in line with your shoulder and hip as far as you safely can, with a sense of both squeezing the muscles and stretching them strongly (this also mitigates the load on the lower back as the legs descend). Remember, your leg only has to drop a few inches below the vertical line above your hips to get things going. And if you're not that strong, a few inches can be enough. In any case, the leg should never reach the floor until the end of the last rep. Nor should it drop so far that the lower back arches off the floor.

    Have patience. Your strength will grow, your range of control will increase and your lower belly and lower back will begin to get to know you on a first name basis.

Your transition from down to up should be smooth. As the leg stretches on the way down to decrease the downward stress, it is even more important to think of pushing the leg out away from the body, using the butt and the back of the thighs as it rises (even more so when lifting both legs—see the following Leg Lifts exercise. Otherwise, the tops of the thighs will have to lift the legs purely by contraction, which can cruelly stress the lower spine—sometimes the upper spine and the neck too—and all them pretty little discs).

7. Now stretch and raise the leg back up to its starting verticality. 10 reps. Twice through. Rotate the leg open from the hip on the second set. Keep that foot strong!

    If you've never really thought about getting your knees straight in leg lifts, the first thing you may notice is how hard the tops of the thighs have to work to stretch the knees completely (the tops of the thighs are actually contracting when you do this). They will get used to it over time and your focus will settle into your core. Flexing your feet and stretching through the back of the legs will help this transition along.

8. To finish, if you safely can, bring the straight leg all the way down to the floor (Photo 57).

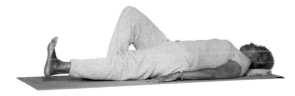

PHOTO 57

If you're injured or unsure, bring the leg down as you brought it up. Bend the knee to the chest, then lower the foot to the floor.

Once again, the degree to which one lowers and lifts the leg depends on one's ability. It may begin with no more than a few inches, but it may eventually cover a full quarter circle.

As always, safety first!

LEG LIFTS

1. These are performed exactly the same as Single-Leg Lifts with two exceptions—the feet and knees should be pressed completely together, forming one stable unit, and both feet leave the ground (Photo 58).

The flexibly challenged and the larger-waisted among us, however, may have trouble getting their legs vertical, without rolling their lower backs up from the floor (not recommended here), which can greatly stress the lower spine. In such cases, though they can still lift their legs, neither comfort nor rest can be found. With their lower backs and butts down, it can be a struggle to hold their legs up at all.

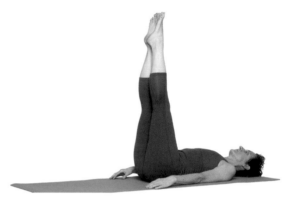

PHOTO 58

To reach that oasis above the center of gravity, such students must seek a more sinuous or digestible path. Until their slendering journey is complete, holding their bent knees up may prove more burdensome than beneficent.

2. Something that will help in all of this, a very rewarding aspect of leg lifts that virtually no one ever seems to address, is the use of the feet and the angle of rotation in the legs (from the hips) as you work. Definition, control, sensitivity and stability can all be greatly enhanced throughout the butt and legs down to the very bottom of the abdominal muscle where the thighs meet the pelvis on those diagonal lines—by their thoughtful use and application.

Once your legs are vertical, try pointing your feet as you take your legs down and up. Try with flexed feet. Notice the difference? Try pointing on the way down and flexing on the way up.

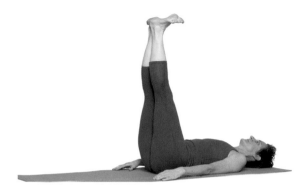

PHOTO 59

Now, in the ready position, try flexing your feet, squeezing your butt, rotating your knees and toes open (keep the heels pressing against each other) to try and make your calves touch (Photo 59).

Lower them in that position, reaching out long through the heels and inner thighs and the backs of the legs as you go down (Photo 60).

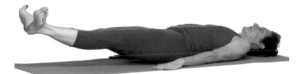

PHOTO 60

At the bottom, point the feet, rotate the knees forward and lift the legs back up (Photo 61).

If you liked that, try it in slow motion.

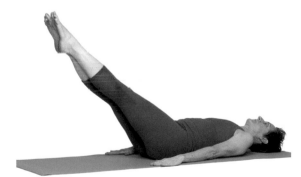

PHOTO 61

Remember, unless you've specifically trained for it, never bring your feet all the way to the floor during leg lifts. Even an inch off the floor is considerably safer for your lower back. And never let any part of your working apparatus relax during the course of execution.

For many of us, good form in **Leg Lifts** takes time to acquire (it sure did for me!). Still, with a patient and thoughtful approach, they can be practiced with safety. When done with good form, Leg Lifts are safe. Done with bad form, they can crush your lower back.

ROTATIONS

The straight forward and straight back motion of Sit-ups and leg lifts will only take you so far. To assist in flattening (tightening) your front, to trim and tighten the sides and waist, to secure the blessings of mobility for ourselves and our posteriors, some twisting of the torso (rotational exercise) should be involved. It can be done crunching, sitting up and in all kinds of whole-body movements.

However, rotational exercises must be thought through. Twisting from the waist is not the same as turning from the hips (there are exercises for both).

To twist from the waist, the muscles in the torso stretch and contract.

The upper body performs this task—rotating side to side—while the lower body (hips, legs and feet) supplies a nearly rigid stability.

When turning from the hips, the muscles in the torso work as stabilizers to keep the trunk solidly aligned with the turning hips. This focuses on whole-body stability with the whole body changing direction as one unit.

Both are great and both will strengthen your waist. Though turning from the hips actually has more practical use in daily life, a trimmer waistline will be achieved by working the waist and hips separately (have a look at samba dancers). If you want to trim as well as strengthen your waist, torso rotations will help you out.

Once again, however you do them—standing, kneeling, on your butt or lying down—form is essential for the right results. These things must be thought through.

One safe and effective rotational exercise is something I call **Crossover Crunches**. It involves working the trunk toward the hips diagonally, opposite shoulder to opposite hip, across the vertical midline of the body.

CROSSOVER CRUNCHES

1. The starting form is the same as for Crunches (steps 1 and 2) (Photo 62).

2. The crunch itself is performed the same as for Crunches (step 3), with one critical alteration: the angle of the crunch. Determine a straight line from one shoulder down to the opposite hip and, when you curl, curl along that diagonal line, as if to draw one to the other. Keep in mind that the shoulder in question is a reference point from which to guide the greater movement of the torso.

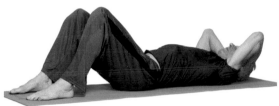

PHOTO 62

The shoulder remains secured in its position. At no time does one pull with it or rotate it forward. Rotation is generated from the trunk itself.

Beginning simultaneously, in sync with your rising torso, pull the opposite knee up toward your chest. If you don't turn your head (and there's no need to), the knee will come toward your nose and the leading elbow will aim down the middle of your hips (Photo 63).

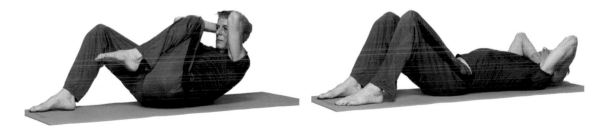

PHOTO 63

PHOTO 64

3. Open down to the floor. Be sure the back of the head reaches the ground (Photo 64).

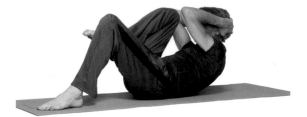

4. Curl up to the other side, drawing in the opposite knee (Photo 65).

    Roll down and repeat. (With one left and one right curl being one repetition, 30 is a good place to start. 50 or 60 make a good regular routine.)

PHOTO 65

Although relatively simple in form, **Crossover Crunches** does require a certain degree of coordination in the body, especially between the bottom of the ribcage and the knees. Try as they might, some folks will not feel comfortable with this exercise at all in the beginning.

The following is an easier, preparatory variation.

CROSSOVER CRUNCH VARIATION

1. Set up as for Crunches (steps 1 and 2)

2. Place one ankle—above the bump on its side—across the opposite knee (which is bent at 90 degrees). Do not put the foot on the knee, as this over-rotates the foot at the ankle. Press the knee open to the side, if possible bringing it perpendicular (90-degree angle) to the body and supporting leg.

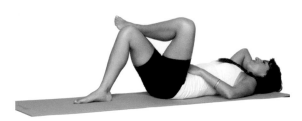

3. Place the opposite hand behind the head. The same side hand should be placed on the side of the belly, with the elbow resting on the floor (Photo 66).
    The elbow supplies extra stability, without being encouraged to push, as it isn't very strong in this position. Also, the arm, folded in, keeps the center of gravity on or near the midline of the body.

PHOTO 66

When the hand is out to the side—as many place it in this exercise—it and the forearm almost invariably push, infringing on the work being done and drawing the center of gravity away from the midline.

4. The supporting foot remains on the floor. The crossing leg remains pressed open. All you do is curl and bring the opposite shoulder toward the crossed leg's hip. A simple move (Photo 67).

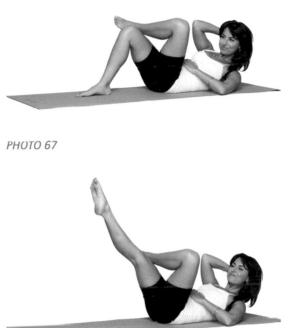

PHOTO 67

The hard part is maintaining the stability of the open knee.

5. Release the curl and do it again. Try at least 10 repetitions. Repeat on the other side. For extra work, hold the last rep at the top of the curl and extend the supporting calf, from the knee, out straight. A simple move (Photo 68). If the thigh doesn't change angle— and it shouldn't—the leg will stretch at approximately 45 degrees.

PHOTO 68

6. Hold your torso up and shoulder crossing to the hip. Do ten reps extending and bending the calf, bringing the foot fully flat on the floor with each bend. After that, if you can, hold the calf extension for a count of ten before lowering the calf and body.

Try these for a week or two and Crossover Crunches will become more accessible.

Speed is beneficial in these exercises. Slow motion will strengthen very thoroughly, but rapid contraction and extension is what really tightens things up, gets that sleek elasticity thing going. To the extent that one can sustain good form and proper alignment—curling shoulder to hip through the belly, never over-rotating the neck (remember, one proceeds on a knee to nose basis)—one should move along at a good clip.

The action of the hips pulling the knees in, in conjunction with the belly curling the body in—as both bend toward the axis—pumps a lot of blood into the muscles, especially when combined with full, controlled, rapid release and stretch. It can really warm the muscles up and get them ready for tougher work to come—providing you move at some effort of speed.

I must address a couple of things here. As anyone who has ever witnessed calisthenics has most likely seen some version of the above exercise, I'd like to clarify my reasons for **Crossover Crunches** specifically as I have described.

First, I did not describe the action of the curl as "bring your elbow to the knee." A commonly used instruction, drawing the elbow to the knee over-rotates the torso at the ribcage, and the line of the curl no longer extends down through the hips (the line cuts short, across the waist at best, usually considerably higher). This thoroughly diminishes the work in the lower abs and sides. It'll make your upper abs strong, presuming you don't strain your back at this degree of rotated stress, but it won't do much for the belly below the line of curl, except maybe let it push out a bit.

This idea can also cause the neck to twist unnecessarily, encouraging soreness in the traps (the *trapezius* muscles) where the neck and shoulder meet at the upper back, as there is usually some unconscious pull from the turning arm and shoulder. The shoulder pulls and turns ahead of the body, overstretches that side of the upper back (possibly straining it or the other side, anywhere from the bottom of the shoulder blade up through the neck) and takes work away from the belly.

Another popular way to do a rotational crunch is the **Bicycle**. Lying on the back, it is very similar to **Crossover Crunches** in general movement (though most people still do the elbow to knee thing). The biggest difference is that the feet remain off the ground throughout, pushing long and away from the body (as pumping a bicycle) rather than bending to the ground. Most participants never stretch their torsos out to the ground, but stay in a quasi-curl continually (not advised training for one's posture).

Keeping the feet in the air and pushing out long, instead of bending the down to the floor, changes a few things. The feet going out, away from the supine body, increases stress on the lower spine, which can cause it to overarch (ouch!) while you're curling. It also tends to work the top of the butt more than the lower and the upper abs much more than the lower. Moreover, without one foot on the ground to help stabilize the spine, there is a measure of wobble—from side to side—in the lower spine as the body and legs extend and contract.

Diminishing this wobble, through strength alone, can be argued by some as a way of building stability—and there may be truth in that, for the right type of spine. For me, however, this **Bicycle** destabilizes the vertical hairline fracture in my lower spinal vertebrae. If I do them two or three days in a row, I will, most likely, collapse in severe pain and find myself unable to stand or walk for days or weeks. (I have worked with others who, for various reasons, find similar difficulties.)

But, that's me. You may find the **Bicycle** beneficial. Just keep a few things in mind: Think shoulder to hip; don't let your knees open wide (rather try to pull them across to the midline, to work the often neglected inner thighs); and extend your torso fully between curls—and take your time. Don't rush them until you've got your form right.

OPEN CROSS-CROSS

This exercise is tough at the beginning, but easy once you get used to it. It helps secure the hips and lower trunk and is especially great for the inner thighs. I have saved it for last of the hips and legs because it takes a bit of flexibility and finesse to really get the benefits.

We've all seen something similar to it: people lying on their backs, hands under their butts, opening and closing their legs. The legs are anywhere from vertical to slightly off the floor, thought the latter of these two seems to be the preferred height. The knees and legs are in varying degrees of stretch and alignment. If the ankles and feet are engaged at all, they are more likely frozen in an unconscious grip rather than thoughtfully activated.

Now, this sort of thing is relatively fine if you're working for discipline—to toughen yourself up, as it were—make those big motors crank—or if you're seeking something specific from this particular form (though I don't know what couldn't be gained more safely another way). You can build some muscle, but I question the degree of the muscular definition that can be achieved and have some concern over ramifications for the muscles in the back, as regards posture and the extent to which the body might learn from the exercise done in this manner.

Let's look at the form piece by piece. If the legs are low to the ground, the lower back is under more pressure to arch. It is harder to squeeze the lower belly in. No matter how hard the belly works, it wants to push out. When the legs open and close, the sides of the lower back, rather than the hips and thighs, pick up most of the work. Although relaxed knees and feet can actually reduce stress on the lower back in this position, they ultimately only exacerbate the shortfall of positive results.

If the legs and feet don't work, the legs don't benefit. If the legs don't work, the hips and trunk don't work as hard (or as thoroughly—there won't be as much refinement in the muscles). If the legs don't work, the body is not learning to think as a whole. You're running the parts but neglecting the function of the machine.

With a few adjustments, however, this exercise can become a thing of beauty and of great relevance to the inner thighs, hips and lower belly.

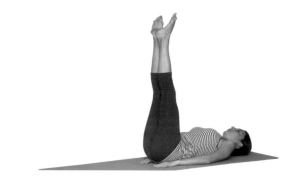

1. Follow steps 1 through 5 for Leg Lifts (p.110).

2. With those legs and feet strong and stretched (Photo 69), open the legs—smoothly and evenly—as wide as they will safely go (Photo 70).

With steady muscular control, reverse direction and draw them back together.

PHOTO 69

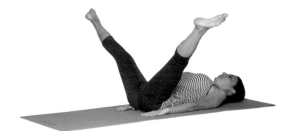

PHOTO 70

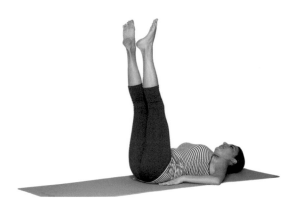

PHOTO 71

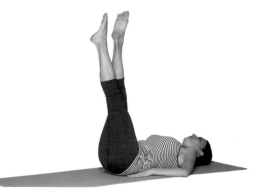

PHOTO 72

The knees may be forward or rotated open from the hips. The feet may be pointed or flexed (beginners will find it easier to stretch the knees with flexed feet). Each variation causes a change in how the working muscles do their jobs.

3. As your legs close, try to cross them with (and at) the thighs (Photo 71), bringing one leg in front, then the other as you reverse the cross (Photo 72). The thighs should actually beat against each other, and the—rigid as steel—stretched legs completely cross from the calves through the feet.

    If the knees are not rotated open, the feet should be pointed to avoid smacking the toes against the crossing heel. If the knees are open, either pointed or flexed feet may be employed, but the most specific work comes with pointed feet. If your pointed foot cramps, try pulling your toes back. If that doesn't fix it, flexing the whole foot should.

4. Go back to step 2 and do it all again. The finest work is found with the legs vertical over the hips, knees rotated open and feet pointed. I would suggest you try this exercise both in the traditional way and in the way I have described. Examine the differences and use them, as you wish, to your best advantage. No more than 16 reps.

ARCHES

Lifting up through the chest and arching into the upper back can have a great tightening effect on the abs. When arching—provided the lower abs are squeezing in and the upper abs are in and lifting—their elasticity becomes more resilient, an effect that carries through very well to daily life. Especially when this activated stretching is alternated—at a reasonable pace—with abdominal contractions (curls), a much flatter (and more flattering) profile can be achieved.

Please understand, though, such movements take time to learn and, done improperly, can cause serious pain and injury. The training for such moves can be found in various sports, dance, gymnastics and mind–body disciplines. A yoga form that incorporates the fundamentals of this movement—the **Cobra**—is comprehensively detailed in chapter VIII, Stretches.

One somewhat safer way to get the benefits of arching into the abs is to use a Swiss ball (also known as a stability ball—and probably half a dozen other names—those big, colorful balls of varying size and resistance) for Crunches, Sit-ups and working across the axis (shoulder to opposite hip). The curve of the ball allows the reclining body to arch between the curls.

However, it can be real tough on your lower back and neck. So be careful.

WORKING THE CHEST, BACK AND SHOULDERS

Presuming a proper foundation in the rest of the body (we'll talk), upper-body work really comes down to two things: what you want to accomplish and working the proper angles with enough weight to get it.

To gain mass—considerably bigger muscles—it will behoove you to lift as heavily as you can (while maintaining a reasonable degree of safety and form) five to seven days a week and eat like a horse (unless, of course, there is a pre-existing overweight issue). The specific numbers of reps, sets, training programs and days per week vary by individual, but to succeed in this type of endeavor requires, in every case, long, hard work and steady dedication.

For most of us, making the most of what we have—toning, tightening, defining, gaining a bit more size in some places and losing some in others—is sufficient. The rules for this are essentially the same as for gaining mass, only you don't have to work as intensely, and you only need to consume enough good, lean nutrition to replenish what you've spent.

Regular, tri-weekly upper-body workouts of about 30 minutes will maintain your upper body just fine. Four or more will make improvements obvious.

As for repetitions, there are some generally accepted rules that work very well. Basically, you should be able to do at least six, but no more than 20. (If you get to 20 and your muscles are not near exhaustion, unless you're recovering from an injury, the weight's not heavy enough.) The idea is to strengthen the muscles and joints without overstressing either.

If you're only pushing out six reps, you're working with some pretty heavy weight relative to your strength. That's fine, but, if you're a beginner, it might be better to save such challenges until you've become used to lifting. Start a bit lighter at, say, the 12 to 15 rep range. (Some may feel more secure starting with 15 to 20 reps.)

There are a lot of gains to be made in these rep counts, and it's safer overall. Starting untrained muscles with too much weight increases the chance of injury and delayed onset muscle soreness (DOMS). This can take days to show up. From my experience, the longer it waits, the worse it hits.

On the other end, going regularly beyond 20 reps can cause repetitive stress pain in the working joints (in this case, from overuse—stretching and bending the joints the same way over and over).

There are exceptions to these rules of repetitions, but the exceptions tend to pursue more particular, specific goals. For most of us, especially the uninitiated, working within this proven format is a safe way to go.

If you're new to lifting, you might be surprised by how heavy the weight feels. Don't worry. If you can safely control the movement, you're fine. Even moderate weight feels heavy to hands not used to lifting.

And remember—heavier weight makes bigger muscle; lighter weight tones and defines. Either way, if you aren't working hard, you're hardly working, and the point of it all becomes rather obscure.

A lot of what you'll see as you improve your upper body will be determined by the angles at which you work your muscles. An easy example is the Bench Press. Performed on a horizontal surface, the lower part of the chest shows the most gain. When done on an incline, the upper chest tends to develop more.

Although the whole chest activates in both, the angle determines the specific focus of the exercise, and the muscle will build in different ways according to the angles used. The width of the hands on the bar is paramount, as this determines which muscles do most of the pressing.

Every part of the movement has an effect. How far the bar is lowered to the chest affects both the working muscles' ability and flexibility. What the back does, how it changes, if it changes, when pressing the weight becomes difficult, has a direct impact on the spine and habitual posture.

When the arms work independently of each other (with dumbbells, bands, etc.), the angles of the elbows, wrists and hands make all the difference. A little change in rotation here and there can have a huge impact on what's being worked and how it develops. And, if you want strong forearms with powerful wrists and fingers, best start thinking about the angles of your wrists and how to use your grip.

One last thing before we look at some exercises. Whenever you're moving heavy weight around with your upper body, no matter what your position—standing, sitting, laying down—your spine, hips, legs and feet are involved. Secondarily, perhaps, but involved. They can help you or harm you.

Be aware. Be very aware.

Generally, when working the upper body, begin with the larger muscle groups and finish with the smaller. As the largest muscles in the upper body are in the upper back, let's start with **lat** (*latissimus dorsi*, to be formal) **Pull-Downs**. (The lats are the big triangular muscles that stretch from the base of the neck across the back of the shoulders to just below the ribcage at the sides of the back.)

LAT PULL-DOWNS

These are best done on a machine dedicated to **Lat Pull-Downs** and **Rows** (rowing). The **Lat Pull-Down** machine specifies the upper back in a way that is hard to mimic. One can get good *latissimus* work from chin-ups and handstand Push-ups (depending on form, of course), but the lats are not targeted the same.

This exercise is performed seated, the weight being pulled down, via cable(s) from above and slightly forward, of the torso. The standard tool used is a wide bar, with downward angled grips at either end. With palms facing forward on the bar, it is drawn down toward the chest, released, then pulled down again. Pretty straightforward move.

Let's break it down.

1. "Performed seated"—what does that mean? Should the feet, ankles, calves and thighs just flop down wherever they happen to land, or would they be better used in securing a solid seat—say, with the thighs opening a bit wider than the hips, knees bent at 90 degrees (vertical above the heels), and the feet aligned with the knees and thighs? Between the feet, knees and butt, this would supply a nice little tripod of solid support for the lower body, as well as building good alignment into the body's memory.

2. How about the back? Upon sitting, does one slump, casually waiting for the pull of the weight overhead to stretch the sagging torso—just hangin, as it were—or might it be better to engage the belly, back and chest, sit up strongly and use the pulling down of the weight to strengthen the solidarity of the trunk and all its contents?
    If the back isn't lifted, the lats aren't getting their work. When pulling down, try inhaling (it's harder, but that's not the reason). Inhaling as you pull down helps lift and expand the upper back and chest into a slight, upward arch aiming toward the lowering bar (alas, they will never meet). Make sure to lift through the top of the chest; don't crunch those spinal discs by arching into the lower back. This will bring a long, healthful stretch to the entire back and help in the fight against those postural gravitational blues.

3. Throughout the exercise—from when you first grip the bar—keep the shoulders securely in place in the (tall and lifted) body. Work from the shoulder sockets, not the neck. The shoulders will get smarter strength, stronger stretch, more individual cut and overall better training if they can remain in a stable position when times are tough.

4. Should the hands grip firmly—the fingers rolling the bar into the palms—or does it make a difference? What's up with that opposable thumb? Are the wrists involved or do they just happen to be in the neighborhood? How one grips, when lifting weights, has a lot to do with the strength and development of the fingers, hands, wrists and forearms.
    When gripping strongly, we tend to focus on the index finger and the opposable thumb—the most naturally secure part of the hold—but in exercise (**Lat Pull-Downs** included), that's rarely the way to go. It works one (the already more aware) side of the forearm a good bit more than the other, which could cause trouble anywhere from the fingers through the shoulders.

An easy way to encourage a full grip is to keep the thumb on the same side of the bar as the fingers—using what's called, in martial arts, a "monkey hand." A firm grip in this manner, with the bar rolled into the palm, will strengthen—and wake up—that side of the forearm that doesn't come first to one's mind.

It will also help align and strengthen the wrists. Few people seem to consider the angle of the hands to the forearms when lifting, but there are great benefits to be had by doing so. For this exercise, the wrists do best when the backs of the hands remain relatively straight extensions of the forearms.

Although monkey hands are not appropriate to every exercise, for those that they are—**Lat Pull-Downs, Rows, Bench Press** (and a few others)—one last advantage is an extra degree of isolation in the muscles being worked.

Once you and your monkey hands are familiar with each other, go back to the opposable thumb grip and use what you've learned. And keep your grip strong and even!

5. The width of the arms is determined by the individual. Generally, the best work comes with the arms slightly wider than a V above the torso (Photo 73)

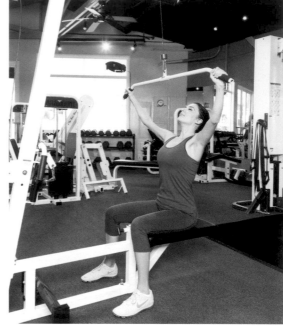

Many people can work from the angled grips at either end of the bar. Some smaller people, however, should not reach that wide. Consider the angle of the arms to the shoulders, the downward and inward pull of the lats and the shoulder blades and find your optimal position.

PHOTO 73

6. Smoothly pull the bar down. The chest lifts tall, arching up toward the descending bar. The elbows bend wide, in line with the bar and the angle of descent (Photo 74).

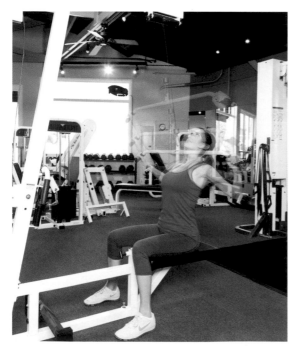

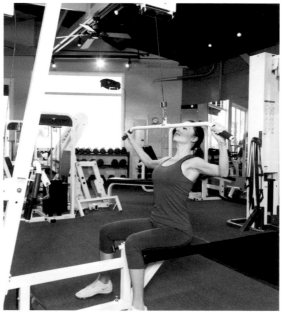

PHOTO 74

Draw the bar toward the base of the throat rather that the chest (Photo 75).

This keeps the line of the pull tracking diagonally through the body, allowing and assisting the chest to remain lifted–and the shoulders down and back–as the bar descends. Both the shoulders and shoulder blades–there's a visceral difference–contract back, down and in, toward the middle of the lower back.

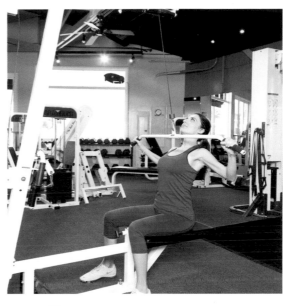

The elbows pass diagonally to the line of the body, from high in front to low behind as they descend (keep them wide). Pulling vertically down or leaving the elbows forward as they lower is an open invitation to engage the neck, round the shoulders, and collapse the chest.

PHOTO 75

Once the weight passes a certain line, somewhere between the chin and the shoulders, the trunk automatically curls in to help push the weight down to the chest. There is no need in this exercise to cross that line. If crossed, the lats hand the heavy work over to the upper traps (the trapezius), the roughly diamond shaped muscle that extends from the back of the neck out to the shoulders and down to the middle of the spine. Engaging the upper traps changes the focus of the exercise, ruins your form, and might awaken various nefarious neck pains and sufferings that are best left undisturbed.

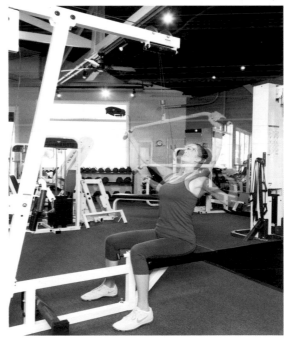

7.   Maintain this slightly arched, solid, and secure form as you release the weight. Six to 20 reps.

Keep the shoulders down throughout. Work from the bottom of the lats and shoulders.

Never let your muscles disengage. Even at full arm extension, keep your shoulders down and back and keep the weight under your complete muscular control.

During this exercise, never hang from the joints—the fingers, wrists, elbows, or shoulders. Disengaging and re-engaging the muscles and joints, with heavy resistance at full extension, stresses the heck out of them.

Aside from the bar used in this exercise, there are numerous other bars and handles available for **Lat Pull-Downs**. Each offers a different way for the muscles to work. Get to know a few.

An exercise diet that regularly includes **Lat Pull-Downs** (and **Rows**—they're up next) goes a long way to ensuring a long and healthy spine and back that will make you happy long into your future.

SEATED UPRIGHT ROWS

Rows are an excellent compliment to **Lat Pull-Downs**. They reinforce the idea of broad, open shoulders, both cutting and strengthening them, and assist in a lifted chest and healthy upper back by training the muscles that pull the shoulder blades toward the spine.

The body mechanics are not that different from **Lat Pull-Downs**, but the angles—and, therefore, the way the muscles work—are. The (cabled) weight is pulled in from forward of the body, at about the height of the waist (virtually perpendicular to the torso).

1. The hands are usually close together, using narrow (6–12 in. apart), vertically angled handles attached to the cable (monkey hands, if you please). The elbows are aligned with the wrists and handles (Photo 76).

2. The feet are placed forward, vertically aligned, about hip-width apart, on the angled platform or bar provided for this purpose. The knees should remain slightly bent throughout.

3. To begin, the body may round forward somewhat, depending on how far forward the handles are from the hips when the weight is first gripped, resting at its base.

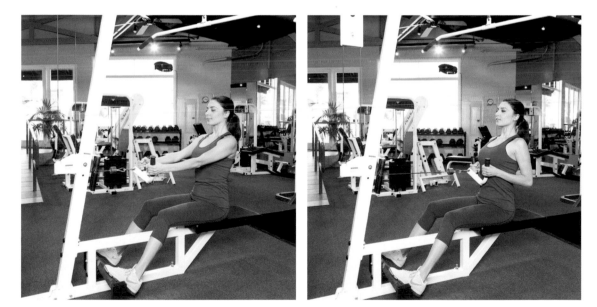

PHOTO 76   PHOTO 77

4. Engage the fingers, wrists, elbows, and shoulders. Engage the belly. Engage the back. Simultaneously squeeze the belly, bend the elbows, pull the shoulders back, and squeeze the shoulder blades together. Lift the torso forward and up against the pull to arch (Photo 77).

The weight draws straight in along the line of pull (pulling it upward, even slightly, will lift the shoulders). Think of the outside edges of the shoulders completing a semicircle behind the upper back. Keep the elbows close to the body and be careful not to overarch.

Maintain an even gaze through a long and lengthened neck.

5. Release, with complete control, until the elbows are almost straight. Keep the shoulders down and back throughout. Try it again. Six to 20 reps.

Be sure to explore and appreciate the role of the abs, lower back, hips, legs and feet in this exercise. Some machines require a long reach forward to grab the weight, as the footrest is well forward of the seat, and the weight, at its base, sits above the footrest.

This allows for some serious trunk work, for squeezing the lower belly into the lower back as you pull with the upper back, shoulders and arms to roll the lengthened torso—rounded forward at some extension (possibly assisted by a little extra bend in the knees)—through a curled contraction, to a tall and straight transition, to a lifted arch, where the contracting shoulders and blades reach their limits above, and slightly behind, the hips. (If the knees did bend a bit extra, they should stretch to nearly straight—listen to your back—as you rise and pull.)

If this type of machine design is available, I highly recommend it. You can get all your regular rowing gains, with some strong whole-body training thrown in. But, you've got to use your legs (weight in the heels, please), and you've got to use your belly. The shoulders cannot be allowed to rise, and you've got to incorporate all this into all that other stuff that is really at the heart of some good rowing fun!

BENCH PRESS

The next biggest muscles of the torso are, not surprisingly, in the chest. They both compliment and equalize the workings of the back. Too much stretch in the back, too tight in the chest (or vice-versa), too much strength in one area relative to the strength of the other—these do you no good.

1. Recline on the bench. Think about what you should do with your legs. (As with **Lat Pull-Downs**, **Rows**, and any exercise performed seated or reclining, your legs and feet have a role to play in the support and structure of your lower back.)

   If the knees are bent much more than 90 degrees, the feet move back toward the hips. This drops the knees below the line of the hips, causing the lower back to arch. The same result can be found when letting the knees flop open or letting the legs stretch out.

   Question is, does this forced arch in your lower back help you in this exercise? A lot of people purposely force an arch into their lower backs when the weight gets heavy on the upward push, thinking that adds strength to their shoulders in their hour of need (it does seem to help, but there's a safer way). I've even seen butts leave the bench in such efforts, pushing high into the arch, leaving only the feet on the floor and the shoulders and head (the chin, of which, is almost invariably poking to the sky) on the bench to support and anchor the move. In this position, the shoulders and back do a lot more of the work than the chest.

   Perhaps a leg alignment similar to **Lat Pull-Downs** would serve best, with an extra thought to keep the knees equal to—or above—the horizontal line of the body. Then, when the upward push of the weight becomes real tough, the lower back—aided by the lower belly—can press (along with the rest of the torso) **into** the bench and get the body weight more behind the push rather than in front of it (which is basically where it goes when the back is arched). No crunched discs, more healthful muscular learning.

2. Grab the weight. The optimal width of the hands to activate the chest is the same as for push-ups. When the arms are bent and a straight line can be drawn across the back from elbow to elbow, the elbows should be bent at 90 degrees, with the hands directly above them.

Monkey hands will isolate the work more than an opposable thumb grip, but one must be careful. When pushing heavy weight vertically, the degree of stress and bend on the wrists, as well as the stability of the moving weight, must be considered.

The weight must be maintained just inside the base of the palms above the wrists. This keeps the weight supported by the bones of the forearms. If the weight rolls down toward the fingers, the finger, hand and forearm muscles can be overstressed and overstretched, and the joints of the wrists themselves can be injured.

Most people new to the Bench Press will find monkey hands too unstable. The idea of all that weight above your reclining body, which could so easily roll off your hands and crush your chest, usually takes a bit of mental adjustment.

It's actually a very stable position, but that's your decision to make. Take your time and, until you're ready to monkey around, keep those thumbs in loyal opposition.

3. The bar should line up, above the chest, somewhere between the nipples and the base of the throat (the higher the line rises toward the neck, the greater the possibility of the traps and upper back taking the load) (Photo 78).

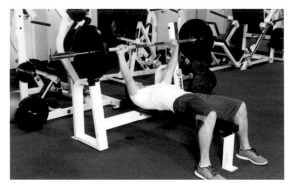
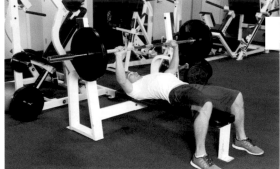

PHOTO 78   PHOTO 79

Inhale as you bend the elbows and lower the weight toward the body (Photo 79).

Lower the bar to your chest as far as you safely can (Photo 80).

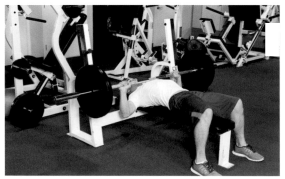

PHOTO 80

The good news about the elbows in the Bench Press is that as long as the shoulders remain in position, the intensity of the work—and the straight bar connecting the arms—gives the elbows little option but to drop, as directly as possible, under the weight. This keeps them in the direct line of movement, protecting their joints and shoulders.

4. Exhale as you begin the transition from down to up. Squeeze your belly and stabilize your body behind the push, keeping the lower back firm and flat into the bench.

    Keep the shoulders down into the torso as you extend those arms. At the top, avoid any of the following: locking the elbows out straight; "popping" the arms out straight by accelerating the last inch or two; and pressing the shoulder forward for an extra push (either upon reaching full arm extension or as a mindless part of the extension itself).

    Throughout the move—down, reverse and up—the weight should move smoothly, under full muscular control, at a speed safely within one's capabilities. The shoulders always remain securely ensconced in the torso. Six to 20 reps.

CHEST FLIES

The **Flies** as named, I have always assumed, is due to the action of opening the arms wide—and closing them—from the shoulders, somewhat similar to the flapping of wings.

What **Flies** do best for your chest could be called detailing. Where the **Bench Press** works the whole chest muscle pretty evenly (moderated by angle of incline and decline), building large, lean muscle, **Flies** work more the center lines and sides of your chest, chiseling definition. Practically, **Flies** help secure the strength and stability of the chest, improve flexibility in the chest and shoulders, and, when done right, reinforce good movement and motor skills throughout the upper body. Use them well.

Though **Chest Flies** may be done in several ways (it's always about the angle of push and the support of the body), classically, they're done on a bench, with dumbbells.

1. Recline on a flat or inclined bench with the angle of the legs and positions of the feet appropriate to support your base. Keep the torso long and squeeze your belly.

2. No monkey hands on this one.
    The dumbbells begin over the chest, arms near full extension (Photo 81).

Above the chest is the least stressful place from which to begin. Beginning with the arms wide, the weights suspended outside the shoulders, makes one initiate the move—from a dead stop, no less—with the muscles at their most stressed and stretched. The top heads of the dumbbells are in line with the shoulders.

The palms may face each other, face the feet or any angle in between. As they open, they may hold their orientation or rotate anywhere within this quarter circle (the direction of the hands will affect the way the working muscles do their job).

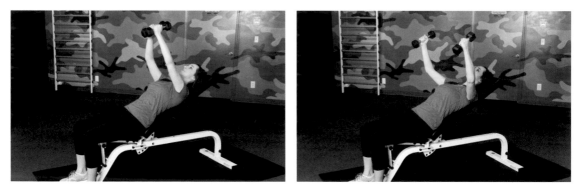

PHOTO 81   PHOTO 82

3. The dumbbells are opened on a purely horizontal line (drawn across the chest) (Photo 82). The hands, at their widest, still continue that same straight line through the chest. How wide the forearms open to the side, is up to the individual. Generally, the wider they go, the harder the chest will work, depending, of course, on the line of movement.

4. Bring them back up along the same line and try again. Six to 20 reps.

    Bending the elbows, however, as the arms open, gives an opportunity for more stretch in the chest and shoulders, as bent elbows can descend farther past the sides, back and bench. (Photo 83).

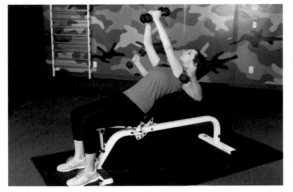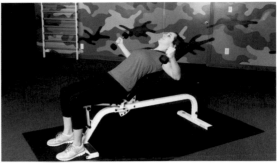

PHOTO 83

Never extend the forearms completely straight when the weight is out to the sides, or in any stressful position. Think about those fingers and hands. Align your wrists. Using these will strongly improve the quality of your work.

There is a natural propensity to drop the elbows toward the hips and let the hands rise in line with the shoulders—forming a W—as the arms widen and descend. This rotates the shoulders to a considerably weaker position just when their strongest load is upon them.

The whole apparatus does best when the elbows are operated directly in line with the movement (at the arms' widest point, viewed from above, one should be able to draw a straight line from each shoulder through each elbow to each wrist). Always consider the line of the move. If the elbow is more than a shade above or below this line—you're looking for pain. Then, when your shoulder(s) eventually begin to bother you, and you're wondering why...

"On that Cold, Bleak, Stygian Night
When Thy Sudden Wisdom and Horror-ed Sight,
Through Eyes Once Merry—Now Sorrowfully Stung-
Realize that the Shadow which Always has Hung
So Threat'ningly Near, so Fright'ning to See
Is Thine Own Silhouetted Monstrosity!

Yet Lift thine Arm—and It Lifts too!
Then "Ouch!"—It Hurts the Same as You!
'Tis Hunched, Distorted, Injured, Worn
And Yours from Mismade Structure Born."*

* My apologies, Mr. Poe.

...you'll know that chest flies are one good place to review for remedy.

The best chest activation I have found in **Chest Flies** is performed with the palms facing each other perfectly throughout (it's hard to resist rotating those palms when the arms go wide). The best overall definition I have found is in a combination of still and rotational moves. The angle of the vertical weight relative to the torso is of utmost importance.

Once again, the wrists and elbows should try to hold the same angle throughout, so the only moving parts are in the shoulders and chest and possibly rotating hands.

REVERSE FLIES

These are usually done lying chest down on an angled bench (45 degrees works best) or standing, bent forward from the hips. Dumbbells are the usual instrument, though other equipment such as cables and bands can be used.

The work involved is primarily intended for the rear delts (the *deltoid* muscles, the chevron shaped, three-headed monsters on the top of your shoulders, above and reaching into the arms) and your *rhomboids* (those which pull your shoulder blades together). Done properly, the entire upper body benefits short term and long term.

1. Standing, face the bench and straddle the seat. Plant the feet on the base of the bench under the seat. Keep the torso long and strong as you drop the hips and chest to the inclined back of the bench; then stretch your legs out straight. The entire body will be in a long, strong diagonal line. When working from a standing position, the feet and legs are responsible for providing a steady and solid base. The feet face forward, wider than the hips. The knees bend slightly and are firmly in line with the balls of the feet.
    The torso will bend forward from the hips with full belly, back and neck support. Keep the back straight throughout.

2. The weights begin together, forward of the chest, arms perpendicular to the diagonal of the body, elbows rounded open, as with Chest Flies (steps 2-5) (Photo 84).

    The hands should line up with the solar plexus (the soft triangle at the bottom of the center of the chest). In this starting position, a slight forward rounding of the upper body is fine. Used correctly, this extra range of motion can offer a little extra. (Used incorrectly, you mess not only with your posture, but the safety of your back as well.)

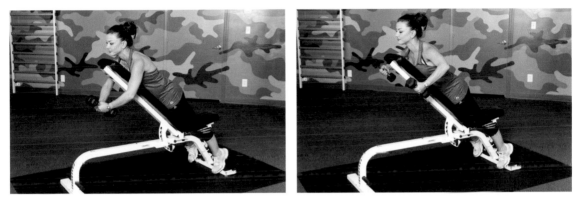

PHOTO 84   *PHOTO 85*

3. The shoulders through the back of the upper arms initiate the move (Photo 85). The shoulders pull around and back as the shoulder blades squeeze toward the spine. The elbows are drawn wide, back and up, on a reverse diagonal to that of the body.

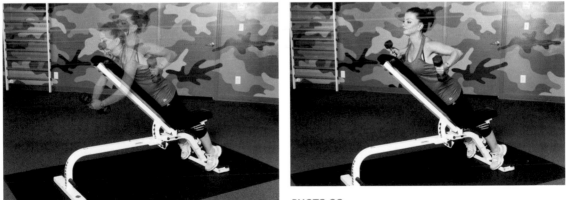

PHOTO 86

The forearms bend freely as the upper arms lift, letting gravity and weight determine their line (Photo 86). **Do not throw the forearms wide from the elbows as you lift** (many do this unconsciously). It distorts the work and threatens the joints. Six to 20 reps.

As you lift, any forward rounding of the upper torso disappears as it stretches to straighten—then arch somewhat—with the movement of the arms.

The back of the neck lifts long, in line with the rest of the spine. Avoid pushing the chest forward and popping the chin out like an angry—or lazy—vulture.

Pull them wide, and unless the weights are relatively light, there will be some dropping of the elbows in toward the hips as they rise. Just keep them rotated open, avoid the W effect and let the forearms (and weights) follow in the elbows' line of movement.

When performed standing, avoid thrusting the hips forward as you lift, and don't jerk the weights back. Use the thighs, hips, belly and back—and the bend of the knees to securely support and achieve the move.

LATERAL RAISES (FLIES)

This lovely exercise is intended for the middle delts, and it is ever so much fun! One can rarely find more searing pain than in this smaller muscle exercise.

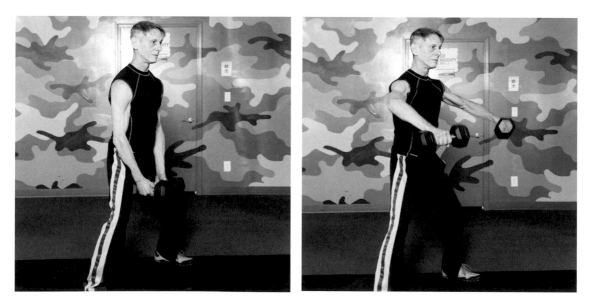

PHOTO 87   PHOTO 88

1. As the name implies, the weights are lifted out to the side from a relatively vertical stance. The feet, legs, hips and torso support as in (standing) **Reverse Flies** (step 1), though the degree of forward bend at the hips is largely determined by the heaviness of the weight.

2. The arms hang vertically (or as close to as possible) from the shoulders. The palms face each other, weights touching. The elbows are rounded open, not strongly bent. Good grip, strong hands, wrists aligned with the forearms (Photo 87).

3. The shoulders and upper arms lift the arms out to the sides, keeping the arms slightly forward of the body throughout (Photo 88).

4. Once at the height of your lift (Photo 89), return along the same line, letting the palms face each other as the weights touch, suspended vertically below the shoulders, and try again. Six to 20 reps.

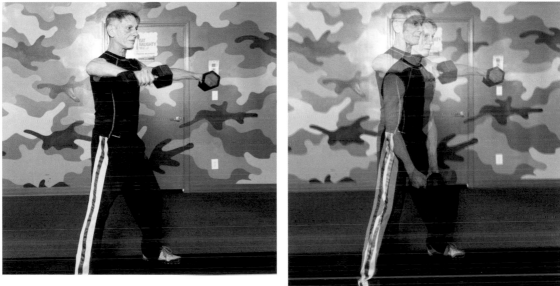

PHOTO 89

Three details are very important to really target the middle delts as you lift:

First, rotate the palms toward the ground as the arms rise.

Second, keep the backs of the elbows forward of the front of the shoulders as they are lifted out to the side. You should be able to turn your head, sight along the front of your shoulder and see the back of the elbow forward of that line. (Do not stretch your elbows as they rise. Set your longest elbow extension at the start and work from there. If anything, the elbows may have to bend a bit as they rise. It just takes a little thought.)

Third, lift from the shoulders first, through the upper arms and elbows. Do not lift from the hands. Let them follow (keep those wrists in line!). Avoid the W (see Chest Flies). Use your body's support properly. Don't throw your hips forward or jerk the weight to lift it.

THE ARMS, WRISTS, HANDS AND FINGERS

Generally speaking, if you actively use your fingers, hands and wrists as you work to other purposes, not only will they get plenty of strength and supple motion, they also often enhance the development of the targeted muscles.

BICEPS (GUNS, BAD BOYS, PUNCH 'N' JUDY) CURLS

I'm guessing we all know what **Biceps Curls** are. Usually done standing—sometimes seated—the elbows bend to draw the hanging weight (in the hands) to the shoulders.

There are, however, a couple of pointers good to keep in mind if you want to get the most work out of your biceps and set a good example for your muscle memory.

1. If standing, the feet face forward—anywhere from together to slightly wider than the hips—knees slightly bent, weight primarily in the heels. Stand tall, support through the belly and back.
    Do not tuck the hips forward when squeezing the lower belly. Think long through the back of the neck, shoulders down (Photo 90).
    The weight (here, a resistance band) hangs at the sides of the body, the elbows not quite fully extended. The palms face forward (turning the palms in toward the body—e.g., **Hammer Curls,** works more to the sides of the upper arms—also a good thing to do, but a different animal). The fingers, hands and wrists are thoughtfully engaged.
    (If sitting or supine, create a solid base with the lower limbs and hips, and lift long through the torso and neck.)

2. The position of the elbows relative to the vertical line from the side of the shoulders to the crest of the hip is very important in **Biceps Curls**. When the elbows are directly below or behind the shoulders, the biceps work less and the shoulders pick up the slack.
    I suggest aligning the elbows slightly forward of the shoulders and pressing them into the sides of the ribcage for stability. This engages the shoulders—and chest—in a very strong stabilizing role, while also increasing the load on the biceps.

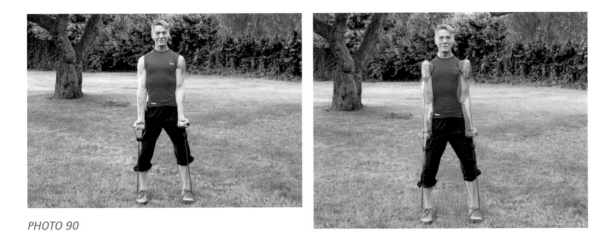

PHOTO 90

3. Curl the weights from the fingers, through the hands and wrists, into the forearms, then through the elbows and up to the shoulders (Photo 91).
    (Active use of the fingers, hands and wrists will additionally specify those biceps as they work, as well as wake up and strengthen all that other stuff.)

4. Control the downward release of the weight (Photo 92)

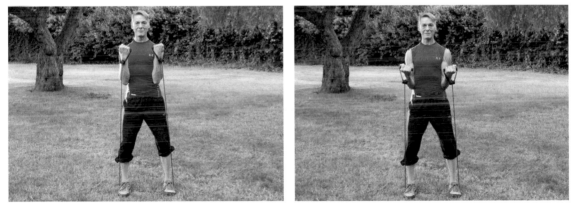

PHOTO 91   PHOTO 92

The elbows never fully extend. Do it again and again and again. Six to 20 reps.

The movement should be smooth, not jerked. There is minimal, if any, rounding of the shoulders and no jutting of the chin. The body does nothing to lighten the load or add momentum to the lifting of the weights. The biceps always take the lead.

Especially when lifting, the actively engaged legs never fully stretch, thus partially precluding the propensity of the pelvis to push (thrust the hips forward) and the belly to pop out.

TRICEPS EXTENSIONS 1

The *triceps* reside on the back of the upper arm. They're the guys so many women hate the jiggle of. There are many standard ways to work them, so a bit of review is in order.

Perhaps the most common form is done, standing or sitting, with the working arm above the head. The weight is bent down and back, from the elbow, lowered toward the torso, and raised again.

1. Align the body as with **Biceps Curls** (step 1). The width of the legs is your call. Extend the working arm vertically, keeping it slightly forward of the body. The weight should hang roughly above and to the side of your forehead (Photo 93).
   (Rather than holding the dumbbell, if that's what you're using, by the handle, try turning your palm skyward and hanging the weight, from its head, in your palm, the handle hanging down between the thumb and forefinger. It's a secure position that will enhance your triceps experience.)

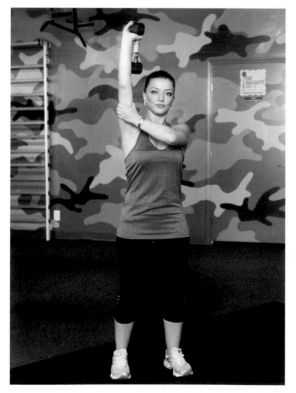

PHOTO 93

2. When lifting the working arm into position, take care to not overarch the upper body or rotate it to the working side. (Both place undue strain in the shoulder, shoulder blade and spine.) To prevent this, keep the elbow of the working (upper) arm visible in your peripheral vision.
   The elbow should face primarily forward. Opening it wide will cause unnecessary joint stress.

3. Stabilize the upper arm by reaching—across the chest, not behind the head—with your other hand to hold the working upper arm in place. Try to not let it move throughout the exercise.

4. As the elbow is bent, allow the forearm to follow its natural path down to the torso (Photo 94).

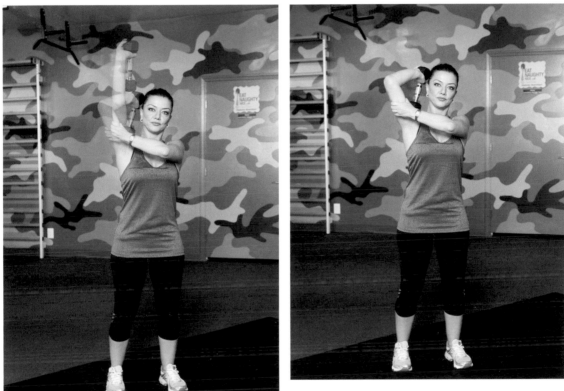

PHOTO 94

Some bend to the base of the neck, some open a bit more to the side. Whatever line of descent the forearm follows, know where it's going and why.

5. Bend that elbow, then stretch it vertically again. Keep the upper arm and shoulder immobile. Work that triceps! Six to 20 reps. Squeeze it at the top (full extension). How many reps can you do?
The knees never stretch. The belly does not sag or push out. The torso is ever strong and straight. The working shoulder never lifts or rotates, but remains solidly in torso firma.

TRICEPS EXTENSION 2

Another common triceps exercise is done, usually standing, arms at the sides, pressing down through the (extending) elbows on a vertical, weighted cable hanging from above, and slightly forward of, the head. Although any number of handles of different configurations are available for cable attachments, I would suggest, in this case, the rope.

1. Align the body as with **Biceps Curls** (step 1). (The weighted cable should be at rest.) With the shoulders in lockdown and the upper arms down or slightly forward, the arms are bent from the elbows to reach the rope (Photo 95).

   Grip the rope firmly with the full hand, as though grabbing a spear or a staff. (Do not just allow your index fingers and thumbs to loop around the wider knobs at the rope's ends.) Use your whole hands on the rope itself, aligning your fingers and wrists.

2. Press your shoulders down and extend the bent forearms downward, squeezing through the back of the upper arms until the arms are completely straight.

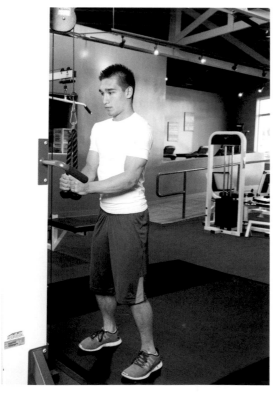
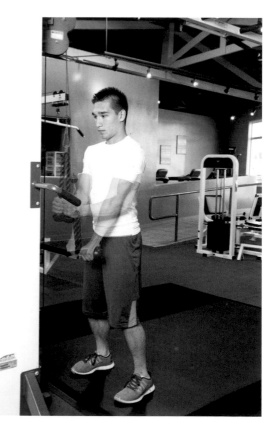

PHOTO 95

3. At full extension, rotate the hands open—to their sides—from the wrists (palms face the body, the wrists remain together) (Photo 96).

Feel the extra squeeze in the triceps.

Use your hands, fingers and wrists throughout. Do not pull the rope wider as you lower it. Keep the hands together in front of the body. Pulling them wide increases the role of the back of the shoulders and diminishes the isolation of the top of the triceps.

4. Avoid stretching your legs all the way; avoid bending forward from the head and shoulders to push down on the weight. Keep your proper alignment and let your arms do the work.

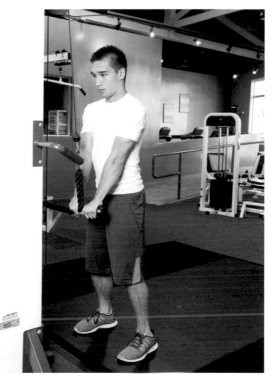

PHOTO 96

5. Return the hands from their rotation, slowly bending the elbows and letting the rope rise. Once engaged in the exercise, avoid letting your upper arms rise with the rope. Keep those elbows secured at your sides.

6. Do it all over again. Six to 20 reps.

There is one more triceps exercise I want to address. It is more complex than the previous examples, as it incorporates the shoulders to an equal extent in the movement. As an exercise, it's great. In rehab, it's even greater.

This jolly little junket goes by the name of **Skull Crushers**, though I'm inclined to give a nod to Rock 'n' Roll and call them **Headbangers**. Whatever's your pleasure is fine with me.

HEADBANGERS (SKULL CRUSHERS)

1. Lie flat on your back on a horizontal bench. Bring your feet up onto the bench. The feet and vertically bent knees are together, and the lower back is flat. If the legs of the bench extend beyond the end of the bench, the crown of the head may need to be extended an inch or two past the end as well (so long as the back of the skull retains the full support of the bench).

2. Using a dumbbell or a weighted bar, begin with the arms at full vertical extension, the weight poised high above the center of your chest (Photo 97).
    (With a weighted bar, keep your hands close together, perhaps Six to 8 inches apart.)
    To use a dumbbell, extend your fingers straight, press them together, and open your thumbs (like a fat L). Place your fingers and the thumb of one hand over the other, creating an enclosed, oval-like opening between them. With palms to the ceiling, the top head of the dumbbell will rest against your palms, while the handle and lower head hang through the opening toward your chest. As with **Triceps Extension 1**, holding the weight in this manner enhances the work to the triceps. Avoid gripping the weight with the fingers.
    The elbows face the feet and do so throughout. Avoid opening them wide.

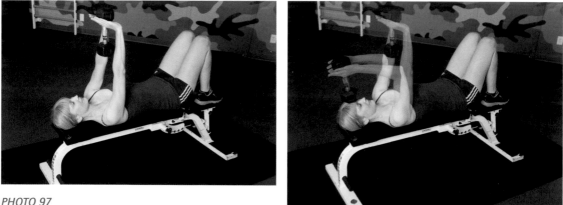

PHOTO 97

3. Bend your elbows and lower the weight to within centimeters of your forehead, specifically.

4. The upper arms stay where they are. Use your shoulders to hold them and bend from the elbows (Photo 98). This may be hard to feel at first, yet absolutely essential to the safety and effectiveness of the exercise. Take your time.

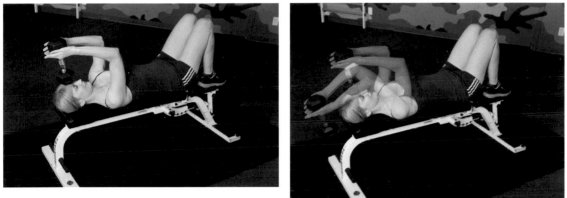

PHOTO 98

5. Hold your elbows at this angle and use your shoulders to drop the upper arms back, behind your head, toward the floor. A little widening of the elbows at this point is normal, but keep them close to the sides of the head. Do not let them open very much (it inhibits ability and endangers the back of the shoulders).

Take the weight as low as your flexibility and control will allow. Think seventh-inning stretch (Photo 99).

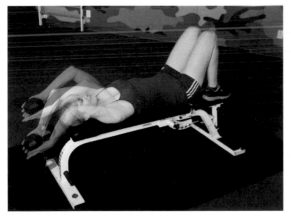
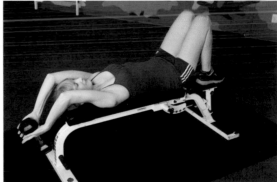

PHOTO 99

6. Without, in any way, pulling from the hands or pushing from (extending) the elbows (once again, absolutely essential to the safety and effectiveness of the exercise), pull your upper arms up, **strictly from the back and shoulders**. (Extending the elbows at this angle—essentially pressing the weight out and away from the head as you struggle to lift it from behind and below—can strain the **** out of your upper back.)

    The upper arms lift along the same line they descended until the elbows have slightly passed the vertical line of the shoulders. The weight, on its way up, will have cleared the head, once again, by centimeters.

7. With the elbows facing the feet—and zero movement from the upper arms—squeeze the triceps to extend the forearms fully overhead, stretching them, at full extension, until the hands are directly above the center of the chest, right back where you started.

8. Continue at your leisure (well, not really leisure...). Control any slight arch that may occur in the lower back when the weight is behind the head, and work safely within your ability. I'd stay with 6 to 10 reps on this one.

There is one more popular triceps exercise, known as Triceps Kickbacks (not shown), that bears review. They are usually performed bent forward from the waist—either standing, possibly supported with the opposite forearm on the forward thigh (one foot front, one foot back)—or with one foot on the ground and the other hand and knee supporting on a bench.

The working upper arm is in line with the bent torso, the weight hangs directly below the bent elbow. The elbow stretches the forearm back, up and out, toward the hips, squeezing the triceps.

If you're working to get tough, this exercise is fine. But, for me, the opportunities for injury or reinforcement of poor postural habits are too great to use it regularly.

It's more stressful on the back and shoulder than it needs to be, and it's harder to maintain good form. Still, if it's the one you like, it's the one you go with. Just watch your form and range of motion.

FINGER, HAND AND WRIST CURLS

There are all kinds of squeeze balls, compression handles and the like to increase one's grip. They're all generally fine, just don't overdo it, and be aware of the amount of pressure being exerted by which fingers and why. Strain some of those long, thin, specialized muscles in the fingers, hands and forearms, and you'll truly appreciate my cautionary note.

Beyond that, there's only one standard exercise I know (outside of skills training—see chapter V, Injury and Recovery) that specifically targets the fingers, hands and wrists. It is usually performed seated.

1. Sit on a bench, using feet and legs, which are somewhat wider than the hips, as support.

2. Using a relatively light weight—you don't want to strain anything—bend the working elbow, palm up, and rest the back of the forearm—at about one-third below the elbow—on the top of the (same-side) thigh, just behind the knee (Photo 100). Place the opposite hand on the opposite thigh for stability and support.
   Rotate the working elbow open to bring the forearm a bit more parallel to the front of the torso (this improves isolation). Avoid rolling the shoulder forward or letting the body slump as you do so.

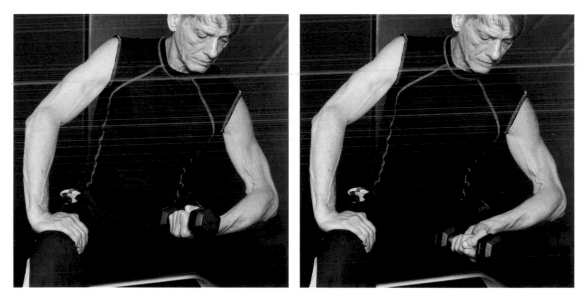

PHOTO 100   PHOTO 101

3. With a firm grip on the dumbbell, roll the wrist open (knuckles drop toward the floor (Photo 101).

At full extension, as the weight drops into the
top of the palm, slowly open the first knuckles of
the fingers (those that attach the fingers to the
hands) and let the weight roll all the way down
into the fingers (Photo 102).

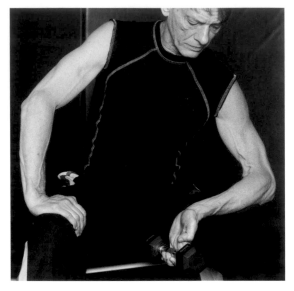

PHOTO 102

4. Maintaining full control at all times, at full
    extension of those first knuckles, reverse
    course and curl the weight back in—first with
    the fingers, up through the palm, then curl
    with the wrist. Curl all the way up, give the
    weight a good squeeze, then roll it slowly
    down again.

    No more than 12 reps.

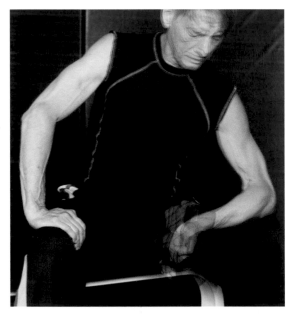

5. Now turn the palm over, toward the floor. Pull the back of the hand up now (Photo 103), then lower to the stretch (Photo 104).

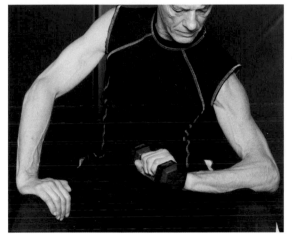

PHOTO 103

PHOTO 104

Do not open the fingers in this reverse position, but rather maintain a strong closed grip throughout.

These two variations may be alternated by reps or done separately. Avoid rotating the elbow back in toward the torso. Avoid stooping, slumping, hunching or otherwise supporting with anything other that a strong, fully aware body. By this time, you may begin to feel that you can see recognizable patterns in the way the body best supports itself in various situations. (For instance, most upper-body exercises performed standing

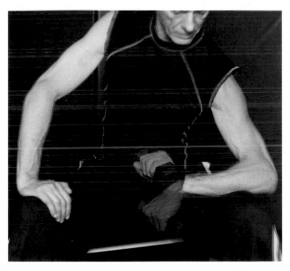

will want to be done with the knees bent to some degree, to avoid unnecessary hunching, thrusting, arching or rotating of the support structure.)

It's not your imagination. Patterns abound in the physical world of your body. They come in both good and bad.

Just as the safe blueprints for virtually any healthful exercise can be drawn from a clear comprehension of the exercises described in this book, so is the same true for flexibility.

Understand the machine, understand the motion.

CHAPTER

VII

CHAPTER VII: FLEXIBILITY

WHY

Flexibility is a wonderful asset to your body. It helps keep your joints moving healthily and sustains your ROM for comfort, ability and fun in your daily life. When maintained together with other exercise, flexibility keeps your muscles and tendons supple and your support structure in better balance. It is great for every part of your body, from your fingers through your toes and even up around your nose (the face has muscles, too, you know).

Though this might be considered common knowledge, what many of us don't seem to realize, until we're much older (I didn't) is flexibility's more subtle aspect: It brings a degree of muscular clarity and sensitivity that becomes invaluable as the decades roll by.

You see, Aging and Gravity are pranksters—Father Time and Mother Nature's unruly offspring. They pick at you, for years, before the myriad subtle signs of your physical deterioration become glaringly apparent. Hour by hour, day after day, Aging and Gravity—aided by their chief excuse, Fatigue—try to drag you down and pull you down in numerous small, mean, invisible ways, with the slow, relentless grind of a glacier.

And, if you're not prepared, they'll get you. Before you know it, you'll find your lower back compressing, arching ever forward and down as the lower belly drops farther into the hips. Or, perhaps, you'll find your hips permanently tucking forward, flattening or even rounding the lower back and forcing a slight bend in the knees (the lower belly still, most likely, plopping out).

As your lower support is compromised, so the upper must follow. If you don't notice the back of your neck slowly collapsing, your chin beginning to jut forward, the slow, incremental roll of your shoulders rounding forward or lifting near the ears in a vain attempt to straighten an uneducated frame; if you can't feel the sinkhole forming in the middle of your chest, or your upper back overarching as your butt seeks out new life forms to the rear, boldly going where no butt has gone before; if you can't be aware of these things and learn to adjust them, you're going to have a hard time maintaining a healthful, pain-free, dynamic posture, much less a well-working body, outside or in.

Regular flexibility training helps you resist these Imperious Imps of Nature. When you're used to feeling long and strong—and know how to make it happen—it's easier to defend against their relentless harassments.

It isn't just about being able to perform that perfect split when you're 25, or reach that top shelf of the cabinet when you're 70. Flexibility done properly offers insight into every aspect of your physically active world. Use it and have a safer, healthier, freer life.

CAUTIONARY TALES

Not all bodies, joints, or stretchers are created equal. The praise (if we're lucky) or the blame (if we're not) lies largely within our genetics, both in how we're made and who, specifically, coughed up the seed money.

Ligaments, tendons and muscles will naturally develop shorter or longer, tighter or looser, weaker or stronger in different individuals.

Having said that, no one need feel trapped in an unuseable form. With the right training and dedication, one's positive aspects can be considerably developed as one's negative aspects are diminished.

When flexibility training is started while one is still growing, the joints themselves can, to some extent, conform to the training and offer a greater ROM. Even as an aging adult's years of problems can often be relieved with just a bit more of a flexible attitude.

In my case, the congenital, vertical hairline fracture in my lower spine—mentioned earlier—came with naturally shorter hamstring muscles. This imbalance created a tight, downward pull on my lower vertebrae, increasing the pressure on my discs and their fault line—making things worse—until I was made aware of the situation and began the lengthy pursuit of enough understanding to relieve it.

Of course, there are limitations to what's possible. For example, the way the bones of the pelvis form has a lot to do with how wide one's legs will safely open side to side. Once the pelvis is fully set, your ultimate width is defined

Some individuals' hips allow their legs to open, if their complete ROM is achieved, to a full 180 degrees. Others, though they spend years working at it, will never achieve that breadth without "forced" stretch (we'll talk), if at all, which can lead to some serious trouble later in life.

At the other end of the spectrum, there are those people who—mostly women (greater natural flexibility)—have joints so loose that, without training a day, they are able to bend themselves into some truly thought provoking positions. However, that does not mean that their muscles are strong, aware or in any way capable of controlling their flexibility. They are as likely to hurt themselves from being too loose as others are from being too tight.

The trick is to figure out how much flexibility you need, add to that how much you want, know your physical possibilities, understand your structural limitations and get busy.

Of course, embarking on a strong flexibility program brings its own set of concerns. During the time it takes for your body to adjust to this new regimen, any number of fun things may come your way.

One of these is a less stable structure. At times looser than you're used to, at times tighter (muscles not used to stretching can tighten excessively overnight), your muscles and joints go through a lot of uncertain territory on their way to a better tomorrow.

This may result in nothing more than some stiff and sore mornings, or it may cause you an injury or two, as you tend to be a bit less in control in these unstable times and may react inefficiently at a moment of sudden physical readjustment (a misstep on a stair, jumping over a puddle, etc.). A new and improved stretching regimen will also reveal hidden muscular imbalances and joint integrity issues that need extra attention (we almost all have them).

As for stretches themselves, they can be helpful or harmful, depending on two things: the angle of stretch in relation to the support of the rest of the body and the quality of the stretching technique.

STRETCHING: ASSISTED, PASSIVE AND ACTIVE

These are the three main avenues of approach to flexibility. Though each can be beneficial, only active stretching brings solid strength and muscular understanding throughout your ROM.

ASSISTED STRETCHING

Assisted stretching is just what it sounds like—there's a Victim and a Perp. The passive Victim is positioned and stretched by the experienced, knowledgeable, safety first-oriented Perp.

Trained professionals are the best way to go. They should:

1. Have an intimate understanding of the stretches they use

2. Be able to assess what you need and safely apply appropriate techniques

3. Know the effect that stretching one muscle will have on the elasticity and awareness of all other muscles in that line of stretch (e.g., stretching the hamstrings [the back of the thigh] can affect everything on the back of the body, from the top of the head to the ends of the toes)

4. Be able to explain what they're doing in a language you can understand, so you can better feel what's being done and, when possible, learn to do it yourself

5. Give you verbal guides, when applicable, along the way, to add your own physical efforts to the stretch being performed (making it a partially active stretch)

ASSISTED HAMSTRING STRETCH

Take an assisted hamstring stretch as an example of making it a partially active stretch.

1. The Victim lies supine on the ground. If the back is tight or delicate, one knee may be bent, vertically, in line with the hips and toes and the foot placed on the ground for additional lower-back support.

2. The Perp lifts the Victim's working leg and presses the bent knee toward the Victim's same-side shoulder (Photo 105).

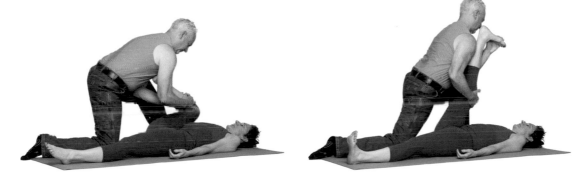

PHOTO 105   PHOTO 106

3. The Perp then stretches the working leg straight and presses it up toward the Victim's shoulder (Photo 106).
    The Victim might be asked to flex or point the foot and toes and press the heel out long and help fully extend the knee to develop strength and control as the stretch is performed.

4. Perps should be aware of how far they can safely go and when—and how—to back off, particular to their body and situation.

To my mind, assisted stretching is best applied when working with the infirm and the clueless. No offence to anyone—I was once physically clueless myself and, in some areas of life, remain clueless to this very day (Can you hear me, Sweetheart?). If one can't physically do it themselves, whether from injury, weakness or a lack of comprehension (remember—**Everyone can learn!**), a little help is a good thing.

When you, as Victim, or your assisting stretcher, as Perp, insist on pushing farther in a stretch, yet your ROM has hit a brick wall, you enter the realm of "forced" stretching. This involves the principle of irresistible force meets immovable object. A volatile formula.

Picture sitting on the floor, knees straight, legs wide as they'll go, feet flexed, heels pressed against the wall. Add someone behind you, their hands at the bottom of your lower back, pushing your hips toward the wall, trying to force your legs to open wider. Whether or not you increase your flexibility, the price could be injured muscles, tendons, ligaments and joints, up to and eventually including hip replacements.

Though many professionals, from ballet to cage fighting, use "forced" stretching techniques, I'm not a fan. The risks outweigh the benefits, if you want a body that will last a lifetime.

There is another form of **assisted stretching**—that of assisting yourself, using bands, towels (to extend one's reach in a stretch and presumably facilitate better results), balls, weights, inversion boards, machines (such as Pilates equipment) and other paraphernalia to "assist" in building a stronger and more flexible you.

As I find these things most beneficial when dealing with injury and pain, you will find my thoughts on them in chapters IX and X, **Injury and Recovery** and **Recovery Techniques**.

PASSIVE STRETCHING

Passive stretching uses gravity to do the work—stretches like sitting in a chair and dropping the torso forward and down, sitting on the floor hanging over the legs, or lying on the floor with your legs up the wall.

No strength is used. One remains completely relaxed and lets gravity do its thing. Passive stretching can be immensely relieving when the body is injured, sore, stiff, fatigued or tense. It also works well in the cool-down phase of a workout.

It's not so good, however, at the beginning of a workout. When used during a warm-up to exercise, all I can say is—what part of "passive" implies that the muscles are getting warmed up? If there is no exertion, there is no increased heart rate. No increased heart rate—no increased blood flow (bringing oxygen and nutrients and all that good stuff) to the muscles. No increased blood flow—the muscles aren't warming up!

Passive stretching is great in the right circumstances. However, when relied upon for general flexibility, it leaves quite a bit to be desired. Passive stretching offers no control over the extending ROM, as the muscles do no work in the stretched position. Nor do they gain strength, positional awareness, or any sense of teamwork.

ACTIVE STRETCHING

Active stretching means you are actively doing all the work. You should work not only the primary muscles being stretched, but everything related to that line of stretch.

Take, for example, the **Assisted Hamstring Stretch**. If you have no assistant, it becomes a straight-ahead **Hamstring Stretch** (see **Reclining Single-Leg Stretch** in chapter VIII, **Stretches**).

Activate your leg muscles. Flexing the foot and toes, pushing the heel out long, strongly extending the back of the leg against the pull of the arms—these build a stretch you can learn from. All the muscles of the leg and foot get more involved as they gain strength, awareness and elasticity throughout the stretch.

And, there's more to consider: the how and where of the fingers that grip the leg; the hands that control the fingers; the arms and elbows that pull the hands; the shoulders that assist the arms; the upper and middle back, the founders of the feast, providing stability for all. Even the non-working leg has a role, to increase the stretch by laying flat or aid stability and relieve a bad back with a vertically bent knee and a foot on the floor. These all have their right places to be architecturally and their right strength to employ mechanically. The back of the neck, the top of the head and the chin should also get involved.

When actively stretching, all the parts that can be beneficially worked should be beneficially worked. It's good for the muscles; it's good for the joints.

Active stretching can be used anytime, except just before bed (the increase in heart rate can wake you up). It's excellent and, I feel, mandatory, as part of a healthful physical routine.

When using active stretching in your warm-up, focus on the bigger muscle groups first. In those stretches that move, use broad, flowing movements through their full ROM. Work from a base of whole-body involvement, at a moderately heart-pumping pace. You will get your blood flowing, your muscles supple and focused, and your mind ready for action.

Active stretching is where the gold lies. It's you taking care of you and getting better at it the more you do it. There's always more to learn.

When you incorporate active stretching into your regular workout, the rewards just keep on flowing. You become the driver on your Highway to Health. Where you go, and how far, is up to you.

WHERE LIES THE DEVIL

Whether you're doing the driving or not, once you're stretching (or being stretched), it becomes helpful to know the rules.

1. How often should you stretch?

2. How far should you stretch?

3. How should a good stretch feel?

4. Should stretches be held statically for a period of time, pulsed or constantly extended?

5. Does it matter which muscles are stretched first?

HOW OFTEN

As I mentioned in chapter V, exercising every day—with the exception of certain bodybuilding routines—is optimal. The same is true for flexibility, preferably building some strength into the muscles as they are stretched. At the very least, one must stretch three times a week for any benefit.

Stretching fewer than three times a week is risky. Your body never gets used to it, and you never gain control of it.

HOW FAR

People begin to feel a stretch as soon as they reach beyond their normal ROM. For most, the sensation begins mildly, steadily rising to a level of discomfort (i.e., pain) proportionate to the increasing resistance of the stretching muscles. Muscles and tendons can be looser or tighter, more elastic or frozen, not just within different individuals, but also at different times, on different days, within each individual (they are, after all, living tissue).

Some feel that a "mild" stretching sensation is enough. If you're new to the field, simply trying to relax, or cool-down from a workout, I might agree. (This is an area where passive stretching can be very accommodating.)

If, however, you're incorporating active stretching into your workout or using assisted stretching to improve your flexibility, mild probably won't do it. One should take the stretch—carefully and continually supported—as far as it feels safe and comfortable to do so. At full extension, there should remain a small amount of perceived pliancy, an assurance that the muscles, though fully challenged, are still alive, secure and calm. If, on the other hand, you feel your muscles have hit a brick wall, you should back off the stretch a bit until your muscles are more willing to accept the idea of extending their range. This occurs with practice.

For those unused to this training, going the full distance right off the bat might be too painful. Muscles not used to stretching can really scream, and pain is a great discourager of continued learning. So start off erring, if you must, on the side of caution.

Too much pain can also cause the rest of the body to tense up, just when it should be releasing static tension to engender the stretch. When the body tenses up, the pain gets worse, and the worsening pain increases tension. This vicious circle can continue until the stretching individual loses all desire to become more flexible.

Releasing tension does not mean that the muscles do not work in the stretch. It simply means that the body remains calm and relaxed while they work. Fluid, strong, moveable, working muscles driven by supportive breathing and a calm mind will achieve exceptionally more than locked, frozen muscles and a body in reactive shock.

Excess tension can cause the shoulders to hunch, the face to contort, the breath to be forcibly held or expelled or any number of negative side effects. It will always cause a breakdown in one's ability, making progress laborious and painful. (Time, concentration, and qualified relaxation are necessary to escape this vicious circle. See chapter IX, **Injury and Recovery**.)

One should stretch to the extent that one feels capable. More than mild, less than discouraging. A positive balance between what the body can do and how much it can stand.

For what it's worth, once you get used to it, stretches that had been excruciating become energizing and, sometimes, actually feel absolutely wonderful.

HOW IT SHOULD FEEL

Well, obviously, a good stretch "hurts," but that's a somewhat misleading term. The stress of a stretch is optimally felt evenly throughout the entire working line of stretch, provided all the muscles being stretched are active or passive to a similar degree. For instance, in the **Reclining Single-Leg Stretch** (chapter VIII, **Stretches**), if the leg is aggressively straightened through the back of the knee, and the foot and toes are aggressively flexed to the same extent, a muscularly well-balanced person on a good day might feel an even stretch from the lower back all the way through the bottom of the feet and toes.

Even for the best of us, though, that doesn't always happen. Something is usually a little tighter than something else. Though the stretch will hopefully be felt throughout the entire working line, one muscle group or another usually dominates the scene. Not necessarily by a lot, but enough to let you know it's a bit tighter than its associates.

And that's fine. That's normal. We do different things every day, our bodies are constantly changing. Ultimately, a good stretch, whether relieving or painful, should feel good. It should feel beneficial.

If one muscle or group is considerably tighter, there's likely an imbalance in the area that needs to be addressed. If one small spot in the line of stretch is particularly stressed, or one thin band of a stretching muscle feels like a tight piece of rope, or as though it were knotting up, or like a rubber band about to snap, or if there is a burning sensation, you've got to be careful. Back off of the stretch a bit. Do only what can be comfortably done (See "The 80% Solution" in chapter X, **Recovery Techniques**).

We don't all feel the same stretch in the same way. Sometimes we don't even feel it in the same muscle group. That doesn't necessarily mean one person or the other has a problem; it just means we can be differently balanced. What we should all feel when stretching, however, is hard, healthful work. It should feel good, but it ought to be tough.

Now, I'm sorry to have to tell y'all this—and keep in mind that I'm a man and therefore automatically tighter—but, in my experience, there is nothing as painful in physical exercise as beginning hard core flexibility training. Unfortunately, that "right" kind of pain is the price of admission.

STATIC, PULSING OR EXTENDING THE STRETCH

STATIC STRETCHING

I don't really like the term "static" in relation to stretching. It implies a motionlessness that could be counterproductive (see the Scavenger's Daughter, a torture device in use in 16th and 17th century Europe).

Even if you hang in one position all day long, there's not much static about it. Each inhale and every exhale affects the stretching process, as does the continued press of gravity. Subtle changes are constant. "Static" just isn't on the playbill. Though I imagine the term will continue to be used, perhaps "held stretch" would be a more accurate phrase.

As suggested by either expression, one gets in the stretch and stays there. The position is then held for a considerable period of time (anywhere from 15-60 seconds, in my experience).

If the stretcher applies strength, the work becomes active stretching. If not, it remains passive.

Some people love holding stretches in this manner and seem to benefit from this approach. Others do not. It's an individual call. If you look into it for yourself, just remember to think, breathe, and be aware of what all your body parts are up to—and why—throughout. Whatever "static" does mean in stretching, it shouldn't mean oblivious.

PULSING

Pulsing in a stretch is an altogether different matter. Though used in choreography by trained professionals, and in the traditional tribal dances of various aboriginal peoples (some very cool stuff!), it's rarely a good idea to repeatedly and rapidly stretch and release the body (or a body part) in a highly stressed position. Just as your head will suddenly jerk upright if it falls to quickly to your chest when you nod off while sitting, your other muscles can also flex and tighten—in an instant—if they perceive too rapid a stretch. Unless you enjoy the searing rip of your own shredding tissue, as your muscles sharply contract in the middle of a surging extension, I'd leave the pulsing to less stressful positions.

(I use the term "pulsing" here, where others might say "bouncing" or "bobbing." These last two imply, to me, anyway, a basically passive experience—a freefall into the muscles' full extension, followed by a bunji-like recoil that throws the moving bits back to the starting point. This is never a good idea for an untrained individual.)

Pulsing suggests a degree of fluid control through the entire working musculature. If you're going to use this motion at all, whatever you choose to call it, maintain control from beginning to end, in both directions and, especially, at the recoil.

EXTENDING THE STRETCH

"Extending" is what stretches ought to do. It's the dictionary definition of stretching. So, yes, when you're in a stretch, you should work on extending the stretch.

Hanging out in mild is not going to do it. Your abilities will rarely even stay the same. Most likely, they will diminish. You must get somewhere near your limit in a stretch to maintain or improve it. Whether working further into the stretch directly, or flexing and stretching related muscles, or passively releasing deeply through your exhale, extending is the name of the game.

WHO'S ON FIRST?

Larger muscles are usually stretched first. You're more familiar with them, they're more familiar with you, and they more greatly control the basic movements of the area being stretched. The back, the shoulders and chest, the front and back of the legs, should each be broadly stretched before you get into any finer work. Once these guys are tuned up and ready for action, you're not only much safer approaching less familiar, less secure, or more dangerous territory, your abilities will be greater for having warmed up the big guns.

If the larger, supporting muscles are not ready, going into a specific, small muscle (group) stretch can effect revelations of a most painful and inhibiting kind. Should you injure yourself while taking such a risk, the frustration level of the setback is enormous.

Believe me, you don't need the pain or the anger. Sometimes, ignorance **is** bliss.

LAYING THE FOUNDATION

When you begin the stretching portion of your workout, first focus your mind and relax your body. Get calm. Then put all your thought into each stretch as it comes along. If your mind is somewhere else—last night's date, what you're having for lunch—you won't get the best available work at hand, and you will increase your chances of injury.

Remember: Specificity rules! Always!

Know what you intend to do and be precise in your execution. A slight rotation here, a little undue relaxation there, and you're in a different stretch altogether. Even something as seemingly simple as hanging over from the waist while standing varies with every change: the degree of width between the legs, the degree of bend in a knee, whether the balls of the feet or the heels are carrying the weight, whether the belly is supporting or hangs. Stretch varies in every slackened belly, every rotated foot, every unreleased neck. Not to mention the angle of the torso (left, right, down the middle).

If you're stretching actively, consider how hard you're working and where. Be sure to spread the load as evenly as possible through your working apparatus. Failure to do so can cause trouble where you least expect it. For instance, if only one finger can reach over the toes in a hamstring stretch, it is not a good idea to pull as hard as you can with that finger. Without the other fingers and the hand solidly engaged, this could easily cause a strain, anywhere from the finger to the shoulder and beyond. Always keep your working bits properly aligned and secured for the job being done.

In confluence, you must be careful not to overstress the areas being stretched. A balance must be maintained between the strength being applied to increase the stretch and the stretching muscles' ability to absorb the pull safely.

Never force a stretch. To whatever extent you work in a position, however much it hurts, it should always feel safe and beneficial. As I've said before, pain comes in both flavors—helpful and harmful—and, for some, it takes a little time to taste the difference.

Don't overdo it. If you're new to flexibility, work your way in easy. Look before you leap. If you're well trained yet wanting more, don't become obsessed. Part of being well trained is understanding patience. Know your healthful limits and respect them.

For what it does for the health and freedom of your physical life, flexibility is a blast. Sometimes an incredibly painful blast, but a blast nevertheless.

So, let's get that countdown going and see how much you can feel.

CHAPTER VIII

CHAPTER VIII: STRETCHES

Unless otherwise specified, the stretches given in this chapter can be done slowly and more passively or faster and more vigorously. If you're cooling down or relaxing for the evening, I suggest the former. If preparing for a workout, the latter is the way to go. (For gentler approaches altogether, see chapter X, **Recovery Techniques**.)

Of course, you don't have to use these stretches at all. There are any number of stretches and variations for every part of the body, and one size doesn't always fit all. However, they are good examples of how to go about stretching, and I have found them to be safe and effective, not only for myself, but for my clients and students as well, for lo, these many years.

I present them in the order in which I use them, usually in preparation for a workout. The standing positions come first, then those seated, reclining and prone. Although my sequencing has arguably been influenced by my background in dance and martial arts, I firmly believe that, when warming up, one should start with easier stretches, and get that blood flowing, before approaching the tougher ones. This way, by the time one gets to the tough stuff, the blood is well pumped and the bigger—and often tighter—muscles are more ready to work.

All stretches should be done at a pace—and within a range of motion—that is safe for the working individual. A gentler stretch, carefully executed with good form, does far more good than a hard pull on a misaligned or unsupported body gripped by tension.

STANDING STRETCHES

WINDMILLS

A well-known exercise seldom analyzed, Windmills are intended to open the shoulders, upper back, and chest through ROM rotation of the arms from the shoulders.

Done properly, they're a great thing. Done poorly, they jeopardize the neck, shoulders, middle back, lower back, knees, and, in tight circumstances, the calves.

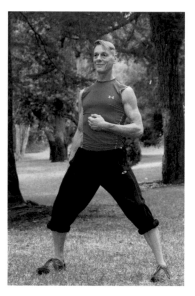

PHOTO 107

1. The body must be grounded and strong. The position assumed is a moderate squat, what in martial arts is known as a "Horse Stance", as it resembles a man astride a horse (Photo 107).

The feet are firmly planted, facing directly forward (to protect the knees, as the primary stress will be front to back). They are one-and-a-half to two times wider than the hips.

The knees are bent at roughly 45 degrees, pressed open from the inner thighs, to align—unwaveringly—over the feet. The weight is distributed on the feet approximately 60 to 40 percent heels to toes (Photo 107).

The standing torso is aligned, as usual, with the lower belly flattened (don't tuck those hips forward), the upper abs lifting into the spine, expanding the breadth of the ribcage, and the shoulders pressed firmly down, capping the structure. The crown of the head is lifted long through the back of the neck.

2. Secure one arm. You may place it at your side, put your hand on your waist or, as I prefer, place the hand on the solar plexus (where the ribs come together at the bottom of the breastbone). Once placed, that arm doesn't move. (If you need the extra stability, you can place the hand on the thigh.)

3. Once aligned and stabilized, swing the working arm forward and up (Photo 108), past the head (Photo 109) back behind the shoulder, around and down (Photo 110), through your full range of motion.

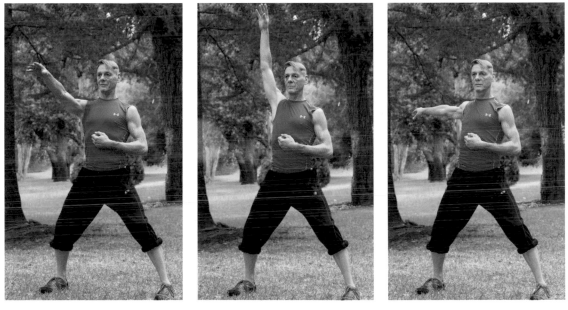

PHOTO 108   PHOTO 109   PHOTO 110

Be careful to keep the shoulder strongly anchored and the rest of the body as still as possible. Properly supported, there is little movement other than the working arm and shoulder. If your body is wobbling like jelly in a hurricane, slow it down and check your support structure. You've got some stabilizing to do. Troubleshoot from the ground up, then double check it from the top down—one body part at a time.

Eight to 12 repetitions should do it. Then go to the other arm. Then, swing both arms simultaneously (Photo 111). Remember, full range of motion. Cross up through the elbows as they swing forward (Photo 112), then up and out (Photo 113), and back and around the sides as far as they'll safely go (Photo 114), then down and around again. Open up that chest!

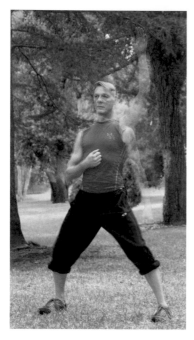

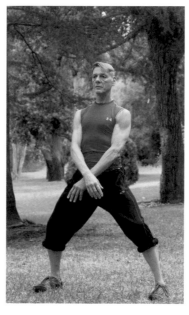

PHOTO 111

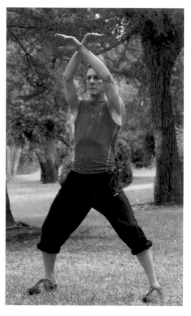

PHOTO 112

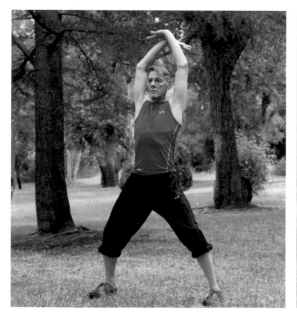

PHOTO 113

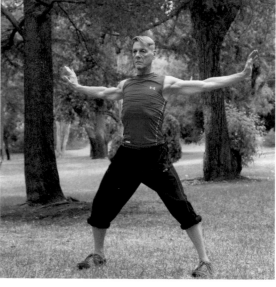

PHOTO 114

4. Now reverse direction with just one arm, then the other, then both. Especially when working in this direction, be careful not to use the torso and shoulder to pull and throw the arm around. Keep your chest lifted and your body still. Tighten your belly and inner thighs.

Always keep the working arm strong. It should never be loose and uncontrolled. Once you're confident that your form is clean and you're comfortable with the move, you can start exploring how the move affects, and can be enhanced by, the reach and positioning of the elbows, wrists, hands, and even fingers. For instance, doing **Windmills** with fingers reaching long brings a different sensitivity—through the entire arm—than performing them with a closed fist.

When warming up, you are depriving yourself if you only think about the joints you're working. Awareness of the entire body is essential if you're going to perform your exercises safely and get the most out of them. Taking all parts of the body into consideration, on any given move, will improve muscular sensitivity throughout the body in that (or those) positions. Apply this idea to all your work and your body will learn how to move fluently in every aspect of your life.

It's all about making connections. Whether in travel, business, high society, love, emotional development or physical acuity, life always turns on the connections.

SIDE TO SIDE

Speaking of turning, this next one involves just that—rotating the body from side to side. Done properly, it offers a good, whole-body stretch from the heel of the back leg through the upper abs and chest, and, for some, through the back of the shoulders and upper arms as well. Done poorly, these benefits diminish, but you'd have to try to hurt yourself on this one.

At the very least, even when the form is lacking, rotating the body from side to side causes a good bit of blood to pump from head to toe and really gets the whole body going.

As this stretch involves movement at several joints, I'm going to break it down into three basic positions that we will then put together.

1. The feet, legs, hips and torso begin the same as for **Windmills**. A nice, strong, supported squat. Throughout the exercise, the torso remains squarely secured to the hips. It will never move on its own, but is turned side to side by the motion of the hips. This immovable square is accomplished by strongly engaged abs and back absorbing the torsional (twisting) forces, while being held firmly in check by the locking down of the shoulders' alignment over the hips.

The arms reach high and away to one side (here, the left) (Photo 115).

2. Initiating with the hips and lower belly, weight on the balls of the feet, simultaneously lift both heels a hair's breadth off the floor and pivot them 45 degrees (Photo 116), passing through a squared center as you continue fluidly, another 45 degrees, stretching your back (left) knee long and pressing your right heel down toward the floor to rotate your hips—and therefore torso—to the right. At the same time, both arms swing—from the shoulders—up to the right (Photo 117). The right knee should not pass the end of the foot.

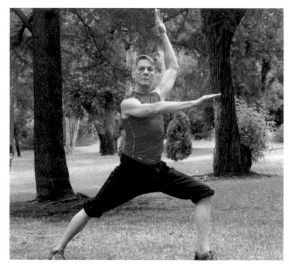

PHOTO 115

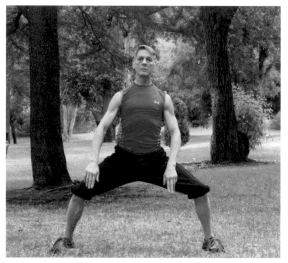

PHOTO 116

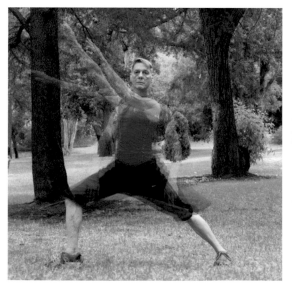

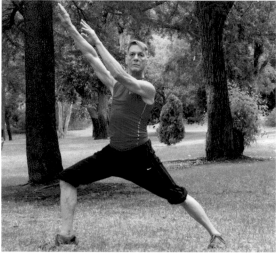

PHOTO 117

As your legs, hips and torso reach this point, your arms, swinging strongly up to the right (from the secured shoulders—think two flinging pendulums), at their end point work in opposition to the stretch of the back heel. As it reaches down and away toward the floor to the left, the arms reach their highest point pulling up to the right, creating a continuous stretch from the bottom of the left heel, up into the butt, through the lower and upper abs, into the chest and the back of the shoulders.

It has been my experience that the best pinnacle of reach for the arms finds the inside (in this case, left) arm reaching vertically behind the head, while the outside (right) arm crosses the body and reaches above the opposite (left) shoulder, bringing the crossing bicep (upper arm) in proximity to the nose.

3. When you reach full extension, swing back the other way. No hesitation, just control. Eight to 12 reps.

Keep your body low throughout, at the same height as the squat you pass through in the center of the move. Resist bobbing up over the middle as you turn or stretching the leading leg as you reach high at the corners.

The most common flaw I see in attempts at this move is the inability to remain low—at the height of the squat—when reaching full rotation. Both knees tend to want to straighten at the end of the turn when only the back leg should stretch—the front stays bent, assuming a greater portion of the body's weight as the lunge is achieved. Straightening both legs not only removes the stretch in the back leg and diminishes the work of the front leg (no more lunge if the leg is straight), it impedes the ability of the knees to square off over the toes as the body passes through the (neutral) squat.

Working from a lunge, one knee is already bent and aligned over the foot, already in position for the squat as one rotates to the other side. With both knees straight, both must bend and drop the body's weight even as they attempt to transition through that perfect squat. A much more complex move.

To really get this exercise down, I would suggest finding the three primary positions in your body, statically, one at a time, while standing before a mirror. Once you like what you see, then begin to work through their transitions until you reach a strong, fluid, secure ability to get the most out of what this stretch has to offer.

So, try to get it right. Keep that body low. We'll do some bending and stretching of both legs together on the next one.

ARM CIRCLES

This stretch is distilled from a martial arts downward strike that is often practiced to break boards in the classroom. However, where force (mass x acceleration, says Mr. Newton) is the focus in martial arts, here we're going for a blood pumping stretch.

You might guess from the name that this stretch bears some similarity to the previous two, and you'd be right. The arms do some big time swinging. They perform the same move as in **Side to Side**, only, in this case, the feet, legs and body don't move. These remain strongly held in a textbook 45-degree squat, while the arms perform a circle of one-and-a-half revolutions in one direction, then the reverse, swinging across the front of the stationary body (sorry, Elvis, no swivel).

The stretch is felt primarily from the hip up through the side of the body and into the back of the upper arm (the triceps muscle) on the side to which the arms have swung and at the top of both shoulders. The downward force of the swings (when done rapidly) is absorbed in the hips and knees, which react like heavy springs, depressing a bit at the bottom of the circle, releasing to the normal squat as the arms rise. Curious? Let's delve deeper.

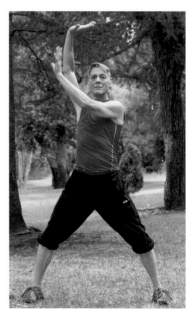

1. It's a pretty straightforward setup with the body—hit that Horse Stance.

2. The right arm begins high up over the back of the head, reaching from the shoulder (Photo 118).
   The elbow bends somewhat. The wrist breaks toward the back of the hand, the inside of the wrist and palm rotate to the sky.

The left arm reaches across the immobile body up to the right, the elbow bending the forearm in and upward to both increase the stretch and keep the weight of the arm closer to the body, which is both safer and more effective in the movement.

PHOTO 118

3. The arms swing down, to the left, across the hips (Photo 119), up left (Photo 120) and around over the head (Photo 121), across the right (Photo 122) and down to the left and up again (Photo 123), to finish with the arms high to the left, one-and-a-half revolutions later, a mirror image of where you began (Photo 124).

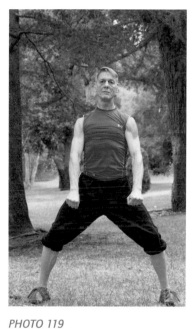

PHOTO 119

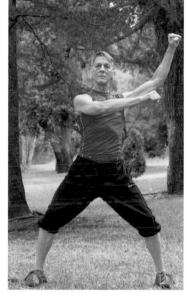

PHOTO 120

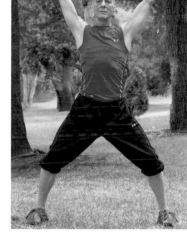

PHOTO 121

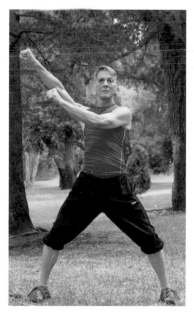

PHOTO 122

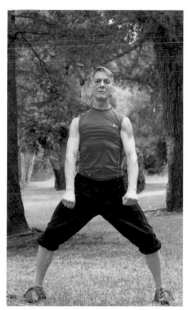

PHOTO 123

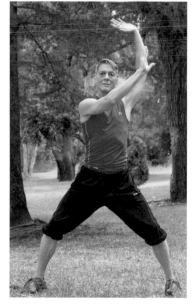

PHOTO 124

The left arm is now high above the back of the head—palm to the sky (it makes a difference)—and the right reaches across the shoulders.

Continue swinging, alternating sides. Do not take your hips to one side or the other. Keep them squarely planted equally over both feet.

Toes are forward; inner thighs guiding the knees. Eight to 12 reps, if you please.

If you want to get all the blood pumping, strength building, coordinative power readily available in this movement, take it as fast as you can—within the limits of safety, of course. Lock those shoulders down, swing those pendulum arms all the way out to the fingers. Everything active and pliable, nothing frozen or floppy.

Use those big, strong springs in the thighs and hips. Feel how they cushion the drop, and speed the arms on their way, increasing your pace and the fluidity of the movement.

Keep the weight primarily in the heels. And, for goodness sake, squeeze that lower belly.

LEG SWINGS

Although I use the word "swing" in this exercise, and swinging is involved, I must point out one important difference from the various arm swings shown previously. Where the swinging elbows were seldom, if ever, entirely straight, here the knee of the swinging leg should never bend, not even a little.

These **Leg Swings** can be performed to the front, back and side, and that is the order in which I suggest they be done. To the front is easiest, to the side is more technically difficult—especially for the standing knee—to the back is more stressful on the standing leg inner thigh and the lower back.

These movements are powered by the hips and thighs, not the knees and feet.

TO THE FRONT

When the working leg is behind the body, the stretch will be felt primarily from the bottom of the foot up into the back of the calf. When the working leg is forward of the body, the stretch should be mostly in the back of the working thigh, its accompanying buttock and the lower back. Of course, the tighter you are, the more areas that can be affected.

As most people balance better standing on their right leg, we'll start by working the left.

1. Stand up tall, feet together, toes forward. Hands can be at the waist, in front of the shoulders with elbows at the ribs (a boxing triangle) (Photo 125), or with arms reaching out to the side. Taking care to keep the weight of the body on the right foot—60:40 heel to toe—simultaneously bend the right knee directly down over the right foot—don't let it fall behind that heel—and reach back with a straight left leg into a moderate lunge.

In order to achieve this posture, the hips must remain forward, working vertically, up and down over the standing heel, rather than dropping back and then lifting forward again with the working leg. The back heel is vertically aligned—it may or may not reach the ground—the straight back knee faces the ground and there is very little weight on the back foot.

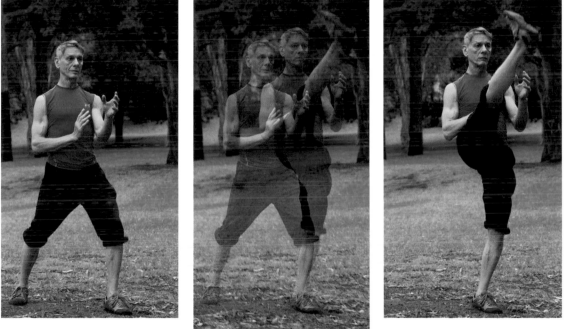

PHOTO 125   *PHOTO 126*

2. Strongly flex the back foot and push the straight back leg forward, using the buttocks and back of the leg (the flexed foot will help you feel this). Straighten the standing leg to make room as it moves. Press the back leg as rapidly as possible through the expanding space created by the rising hips.

   As the standing leg reaches its full height, the flexed foot of the straight working leg passes under the hips and is thrown quickly forward and out, causing it to rise (by reason of its being anchored at the hip) (Photo 126).

3. When that strong, straight, forward lifting missile has reached its upward limit, it rapidly is returned—down and back with a straight knee all the way—to the rear lunge position. The moment it passes under the hip, the standing leg begins to bend again to the lunge.

4. Eight to 12 repetitions, each side.

Keep your torso tall, lifted, and squared throughout, with shoulders stabilized. The four greatest technical challenges seem to be

1. maintaining the weight over the standing leg and foot when the working leg goes to the back;

2. keeping the standing heel on the ground and the standing leg and lower back straight, when the working leg is at its highest point forward;

3. maintaining a straight working knee throughout the exercise; and

4. causing the working leg to lift forward from the muscles of the butt and back of the leg, instead of pulling it up from the knee and top of the thigh.

TO THE BACK

This stretch should not be done unless one has something stable to hold on to with the hands (the back of a chair, a secured horizontal bar, that sort of thing). It is important that there be room for the head and shoulders to drop above, or slightly in front of, the hands when the body is bent forward at the waist.

The main stretch comes in the thigh of the standing leg.

1. Stand up tall, feet together, toes slightly open. With the shoulders over the hips and the hips over the standing leg, place your hands on the stabilizing surface and extend the working leg forward as you stretch (point) the foot (Photo 127). Take the leg forward (from the socket—no forward movement in the hips!) until only the ends of the toes remain in contact with the ground.

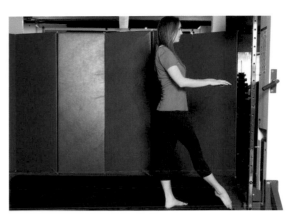

PHOTO 127

2. Using your standing hip as the fulcrum, pull the working leg in, flexing the foot by degrees to trim the leg's length as it approaches the hip.

3. As it passes under the hip, throw it back and up with a strong, straight knee. This action will bend the torso forward from the hips as the working leg climbs higher (Photo 128). Keep your torso firm, shoulders in place. The head remains level, the face straight forward. Take care not to jut your chin out or roll your shoulders forward, and that belly better be squeezing.

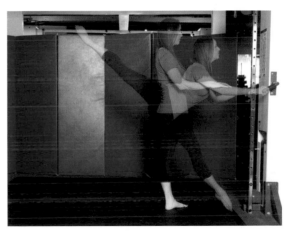

4. To return, the spine lifts, initiating from the head and shoulders, through the fulcrum of the hips, causing the firmly stretched leg to lower. The leg then passes under the hip to point the foot to the front and do it all over again.

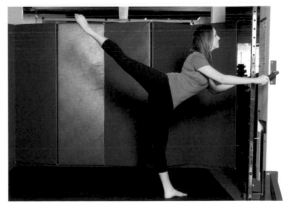

5. Do 8 to 12 repetitions, each side.

PHOTO 128

As the leg swings to the back, there is a desire in a tighter or less trained body to twist the torso, from the hips, open to the working leg side, to ease the stress of the stretch. This cuts down the benefits and increases the risk of injury, especially to the lower back and the standing hip and thigh.

TO THE SIDE

Though grouped here with the other leg swings, this one should be saved until the hips and lower-back have been well—and actively—stretched.

Generally done free standing, if you're new to this sort of thing, I would suggest holding on to a horizontal, stabilized bar or chair, paralleling your standing leg side. The elbow should remain relaxed and slightly forward of the shoulder to prevent twisting the torso.

The stretch is found underneath and inside the working thigh and in the hips and lower back as well.

1. Stand tall, feet together, toes slightly open. Arms are open to the sides at shoulder height (elbows forward of the shoulders), or the hands may be on the waist.

    With as little rotation as possible in the torso (shoulders, at least, should stay square to the front), step across and behind the standing leg with the working leg (much as a woman might begin a formal curtsy, but with strength). Place the working leg in a diagonal lunge (Photo 129).

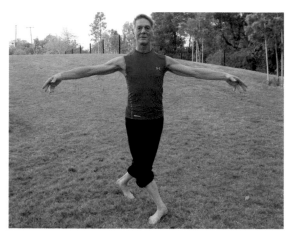

PHOTO 129

As in **Leg Swings** to the front and back, the weight remains predominantly on the standing foot. When the working leg is in a diagonal lunge to the back, the working knee may soften or even bend the slightest touch, to make you more comfy. However, when the working leg is forward of the body—up and out to the side—the standing leg must be straight.

2. As in **To the Front**—although in this case diagonally—the working leg is pressed past the hip as the standing leg straightens.

   It passes from across and behind the standing leg to fire diagonally out and up toward the corner of the room on the working-leg side, roughly 45 degrees to the torso and hips (Photo 130).

3. Once there, it returns to the lunge and repeats the process 8 to 12 times.

   The big danger in this exercise is misalignment of the standing knee. In the lunge position, the standing foot, being turned open (to the outside of the body, to accommodate the squaring of the hips and shoulders when the working leg is forward and out), is in direct opposition to the hips, which may rotate in the opposite direction as the working foot crosses behind the standing leg.

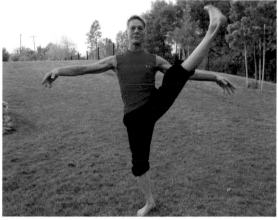

PHOTO 130

This puts the alignment of the standing leg in a spiral. In this situation, the (bent) standing knee may not line up exactly with the ball of the foot. It will rotate open, but perhaps not quite as far as the foot. It forms a balanced bridge (connection) between the two opposing forces of foot and hip rotation.

Without constant attention, working on such a spiral can easily tweak that knee. So, pay attention. Distribute the body's weight evenly through the standing foot (don't put the weight in the toes—keep that heel down and strong).

If you feel stress in the knee, either twisting or under the kneecap, go back to the beginning and check your form. Maybe you aren't ready to turn the standing foot that far open. Maybe your knee is too far forward. Maybe you're not rotating it from the hip or supporting with your lower belly.

Take your time. Get it right. Work out that rotation. Hold on to something as long as you need to (I certainly did).

BENDING AND STRETCHING (USING THE KNEES AND HIPS)

This is a series of stretches done standing, with the torso bending forward and down, belly supporting, and the hands firmly on the floor. These stretches benefit the lower and upper back, shoulders and neck, the inner and back of the thighs, the hips, the calves, ankles and feet.

Though the primary focus of each stretch is the lower back, the primary stretch one feels changes by position and individual.

FEET WIDE, TOES FORWARD

1. The feet are no more than twice as wide as the hips. Stand tall and begin rolling the body forward and down, starting from the top of the head. Move smoothly and evenly and support with the belly. Let the knees bend, as necessary, to place the hands on the floor (Photo 131).
    Remember to maintain the weight in your heels and keep them firmly on the floor. Avoid stressing your knees by getting out over your toes. If you don't have the flexibility to reach the floor with good form, a higher surface (low bench, stack of books, etc.) may be used for the hands. To get the benefits and remain safe, the hands must be solidly in touch with the supporting surface, as they assist in the stability and control of the movement.

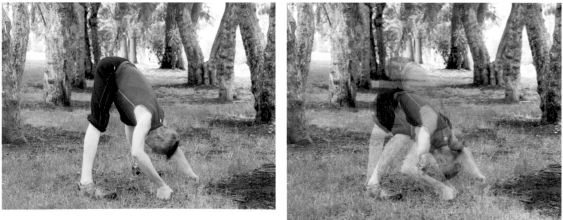

PHOTO 131

2. With the neck completely relaxed (a lot of people have trouble with that one, as I did in the above photo), bend your knees and take the top of your head toward the floor.

Get it as close to the floor as you can (the elbows must bend to allow for this) (Photo 132).

3. Try to keep your head down there while you stretch the knees and straighten the legs. Feels good, doesn't it?

4. Eight to 12 reps, if you please.

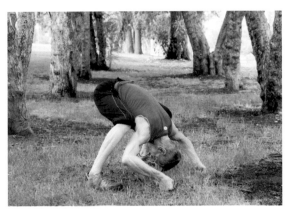

PHOTO 132

While this movement appears to be very straightforward, without attention to detail there is as much opportunity for injury as there is for improvement.

Pay attention to your neck. Pay attention to your belly (to support the lower back). Watch the alignment of the knees with the feet (from the inner thighs, if you please) and the distribution of weight in the feet. Scrutinize all your form and do your best to get it right.

A variation of this stretch can be achieved by doing nothing more than focusing on how low the hips will bend instead of focusing on putting the top of the head on the floor. (There is a point where the head will go no further, but the hips might.)

Lowering the hips beyond this point stretches further into the lower back, butt and upper thighs. It can feel very nice, but it also puts a lot of stress in the lower back. If you're not ready for it, this stretch can overwhelm that area and thoroughly unhappy your camper experience.

In an uninjured body, taking the head to the floor is always safer than taking the hips to their lowest point.

UP ON THE TOES

1. This exercise is identical to the previous one with the exception of the feet. In this one, the heels are strongly raised throughout (this builds strength in the whole apparatus when the knees are straightest and especially in the feet, ankles and knees when the knees are bent).

2. As the knees bend, press the heels to their highest point possible. Watch your alignment. Put the weight of the body firmly in the balls of the feet (Photo 133). Don't let those ankles roll open!

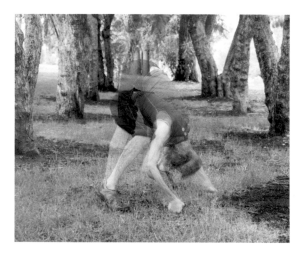 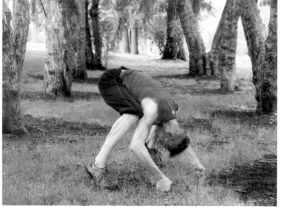

PHOTO 133

If the weight goes onto the toes, your knees—and therefore bodyweight—has shifted too far forward.

3. Try to keep the heels high and straighten the knees as far as possible, with the hands firmly supported on the floor (Photo 134).

Use that belly. Relax that neck. Do 8 to 12 repetitions.

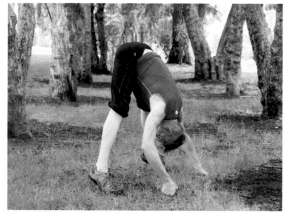

PHOTO 134

RIGHT AND LEFT

1. From the position you've just achieved, return the heels to the floor and redistribute the body's weight evenly through the foot.

2. Reach over and grip the back of one leg (preferably below the knee, as low as you can), and pull your bent torso in toward the front of that leg (Photo 135). Think chest toward the front of the knee.

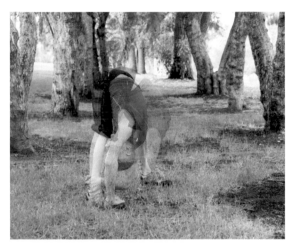 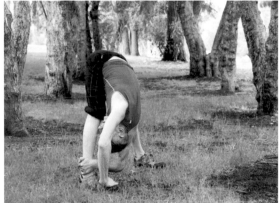

PHOTO 135

3. Get a nice stretch before shifting to the other leg.

Easier variations: Turn the feet, which should be pointing directly forward, open to the side; bring the torso down just outside of the leg, instead of straight in to the front.

WALKING THE FEET TOGETHER

1. From your position, bring the torso back to center and again place the hands on the floor for added support.

2. Using the rotation from the thighs at the hips, turn the toes of both feet open equally (Photo 136). The knees, of course, will open to the same line.

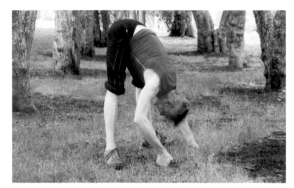

PHOTO 136

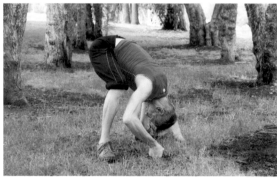

PHOTO 137

3. Bend the knees—good alignment over the balls of the feet, please—with the intention of getting the top of the head to the floor (Photo 137).

4. Keep the torso as low as possible and stretch the knees. At their highest point, keep the heels where they are and, again using rotation from the hips, turn the knees and toes in as far as you can (Photo 138).

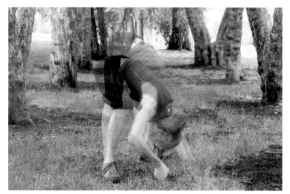

5. Bend and stretch in this position, keeping that torso low.
    At the hips' highest point, leave the toes where they are and turn the heels in, again exclusively from the hips.

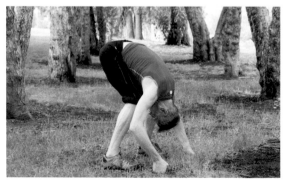

PHOTO 138

6. You are now in the same position as step 2 (Photo 136) previously, only the feet are closer together and the angle of stretch is more acute.

   Bend and stretch here, then continue bending and stretching, walking the feet in, heels and toes alternately, both open and pigeon-toed, until the feet are all the way together.

7. With the feet together, leave the knees slightly bent. Place your palms together at the base of your spine, preferably with fingers interlaced and elbows stretched (a matter of flexibility).

8. Lift your arms as high above your back as you reasonably can (Photo 139).

   Once there, enjoy the stretch before relaxing the arms and letting them fall to the ground.

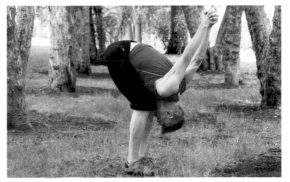

PHOTO 139

9. With the arms on the ground, relax and take a deep breath. As you exhale, squeeze the belly and roll the body up (Photo 140), one vertebra at a time, the head coming up last (Photo 141), until your fully supported verticality has been achieved (Photo 142).

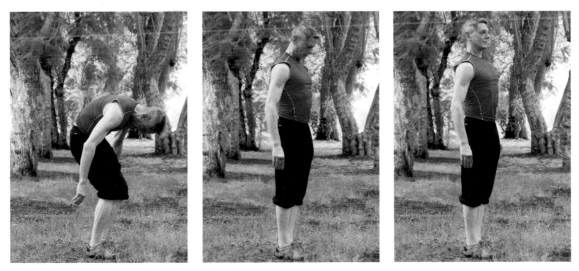

PHOTO 140 *PHOTO 141* *PHOTO 142*

Nice, huh?

SITTING ON THE JOB

Having done some good warming up and stretching of the lower back, hips and back of the legs, it's time to shift focus to the smaller muscles—the inner and outer hips and thighs, the tops of the shoulders and sides of the body—as we increase overall ROM throughout the area.

HALF LOTUS VARIATION

Though similar in starting position to the Lotus of traditional yoga, there are differences, both obvious and subtle, in the way this stretch operates. Please pay attention.

1. Sit on the floor and cross your legs. Lift your back up straight, beginning from the lower back and hips and right on up through the crown of the head.

    If you cannot lift the back up straight on its own, put your butt all the way against the wall—and I mean all the way—no space left in between. Use the wall to support your lower back. This gives you the opportunity to lift the upper back—through the abs, shoulder placement and crown of the head (the back of the head will not quite touch the wall)—and put the entire back vertically flat against the wall. Now cross your legs to the extent that you can.

2. If you have the flexibility, take one foot (let's go with the left) and place it in the crease between the right thigh and calf (Photo 143).

    Do not, as traditional yoga does, place the foot on top of the right thigh. This can strain both the knee, top of the foot and the ankle of the top leg as we move.

    However, if you're too tight, just cross the legs and leave the left foot in front.

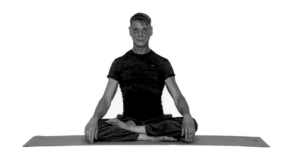

PHOTO 143

3. Take a slow, deep breath, lifting tall through the torso and head. As you exhale, roll the body forward and down—starting from the crown of the head—and walk your hands forward and out (use your fingers) on the floor as the body descends (Photo 144).

The hands—or fingers—walking thusly, gently draw the torso out from the upper back—keep those shoulders in place—as it bends itself ever farther forward from the lower back. This way, the entire structure is stretched, from the fingers, hands, arms and shoulders into the lower spine, butt and inner and outer thighs.

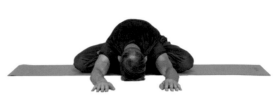

PHOTO 144

4. Once you've gone as far as you're comfortable going, relax your elbows, hands and fingers. You'll find that the friction of the floor against your palms keeps the arms slightly more extended than they would otherwise be when completely relaxed.

5. Inhale deeply. Feel the breath filling the body from way down in the lower back, all the way up through the spine and the muscles of the back, into the shoulders, back of the neck and the crown of the head.

    If you remain completely relaxed, as you exhale—from the top of the head down, through the back and into the hips—your stretch will increase, marginally, from where you began to inhale. Walk your fingers and hands forward on the floor to accommodate the increased forward drop of the body.

    With every deep and even breath, your stretch will increase until you reach your max.

Understand that, if you take your body so far forward that your butt comes off the floor more than an inch or so, you are not increasing your stretch, you're just destabilizing the move and putting more stress in your lower back.

6. This part is on an "if it feels good" basis, which is mostly determined by your degree of flexibility in this position. Feel free to go right on to step 8.

If it feels good to do so, at your maximum stretch, interlace your fingers, invert your palms, and stretch them as far out along the floor (above the head) as you possibly can. If the shoulders maintain their appropriate alignment, a very beneficial finger, wrist, arm, shoulder, and upper-back stretch can be added to the ongoing release in the hips, thighs, and lower back.

7. From your maximum stretch (fingers not entwined), use your hands to lead your torso out and around to the left.

    Keep your right hip on the floor as you go, but work that stretch, from the outreaching hands and arms all the way down to the right hip. Your chest faces the floor until you reach or pass the left knee (Photo 145).

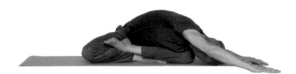

PHOTO 145

As you reach the left knee, place your left forearm and hand—palm down—on the floor, with the elbow vertically under, yet slightly forward of, the left shoulder (the torso is now leaning to the left). The forearm, flat on the floor, roughly follows the angle of the left thigh (this assists the left shoulder in properly aligning as the body is rotated up).

Stabilizing on the hips and left forearm, rotate the right side of your torso up and to the back, opening your face and chest to the front (Photo 146).

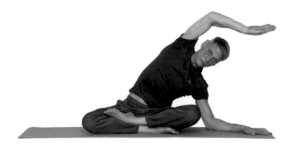

PHOTO 146

If you're tighter, the left elbow may rise at this point, in order to keep the right hip on the floor. Although you are leaning to the left, align the spine vertically over the hips. (If you are sitting against a wall, your back will be flat against that wall.)

The right arm reaches up, over the shoulders and head, and out, along with the torso (flat, against the wall) to the left. The elbow does not straighten, rather it arches strongly, reaching across the top of the head with the inside of the wrist and the palm to the ceiling. Avoid dropping your head forward. Keep your chin in. Everything should remain lifted through that sideways curve.

Keep an eye on your supporting shoulder (at the moment, your left). It will regularly display a propensity to roll forward in this position and must be kept at bay.

Now your body is set. Keep it that way

8. Support with your belly and inhale up into your chest. Stretch your right arm out and, using your right shoulder only (primarily the deltoid muscles—the delts—on the top of the shoulder), press your strong right arm out (Photo 147) and down, to the right (Photo 148).

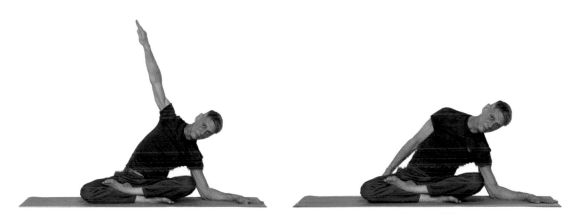

PHOTO 147   PHOTO 148

Stretch the arm out straight as you go. Stretch through the wrists, reach with your fingers, all the way down to the floor.

Upon touching the floor, the arm quickly recoils, up and back, over the head to the left, to repeat the move 8 to 12 times.

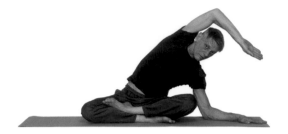

PHOTO 149

9. Finish where you start, at the top, right arm high and to the left (Photo 149).
    Remaining on the hips and left forearm, rotate the right side of your torso forward and down to
    the left, right arm reaching out and down complimentarily, until the torso is again facing the floor
    in the vicinity of the left knee (Photo 150).

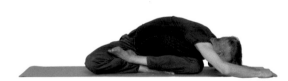

PHOTO 150

Both arms again reach out along the floor to enhance that oh-so-stretchy feeling and keep the back
and hips stable.

Now, just let the fingers do the walking Out on the distant perimeter of the stretch, they lead the
arms and body forward and around to the right, to the neighborhood of the right knee.

At this juncture, return to step 8, just reverse the roles of the arms. Right supports; left swings.

10. No, that's not all. After you've completed steps 1 through 8, change your legs to put the right leg on top, or in front of the left if they're just crossed, and do it all over again. This time, after stretching forward, the body will begin moving first to the right.

If you feel pain in one knee or the other, decrease its bend and moderate the stretch.

Although I have only experienced this once in thousands of uses, there was one time I proceeded, from the first forward stretch, to take my torso to the lower leg side (or inner, if they're just crossed) before going to the upper (the one whose foot rests in the other's crease). I had often done this indiscriminately in the past but, on this occasion, I fell victim to a severe burning pain on a particular part of my upper knee.

I recognized that the upper knee is under greater rotational stress throughout the exercise and determined, in the future, to always turn to the upper knee first. Since that time, I have never again had the questionable pleasure of that particular cause of pain.

FLUTTER-BYS

I never really cared for the term **Butterflies**, by which most folks who grew up in a gym know this next position. Where I studied, it was always "soles of the feet together"—efficient, descriptive, but also kinda clunky.

So I've settled with **Flutter Bys**, drawn from the writings of Lewis Carroll, who, if I'm not mistaken, observed that "butterflies flutter by"...though I could be wrong.

Calling these little hip rippers **Flutter Bys** reminds me not to take things too seriously (when better to kick back and have a laugh than when your inner thighs are being torn from your body?). And the phrase is close enough to **Butterflies** for gym rodents (I don't want to say "rats"—sounds impolite) to figure out.

Yet, perhaps, it is also a phrase distant enough to remind one that, unlike your run of the mill **Butterflies**, this stretch comes with several specifics which, though seldom taught, make these little darlins so much more painful and effective.

As with the **Half Lotus Variation**, the beginning of this stretch focuses on the hips and lower back. However, the inner thighs and entire backs of the legs, and the feet, soon join the party.

Shall we dance?

1. Sit with the soles of the feet together. Draw them toward your hips as you bend and open your knees, as far as possible to the sides.

2. Grab your ankles by placing two fingers above and two fingers below the bony bumps on the outside of your ankles (Photo 151). This allows the fingers room to grip the calf and foot without being overly mashed into the floor when the knees are at their widest (a mat also helps). The thumbs wrap over the top of the calves to grip inside.

Unfortunately, almost all people, in this position, pull their bodies lower by latching on to the front half of their feet. Pulling from the feet in this way turns and rotates the feet to the inside, something they are already inclined to do.

When one adds the regular stress of pulling to this inward inclination, it reinforces the ankles' default to this position and can lead to weakening, overstretching and otherwise destabilizing the outside of the ankles, the very area that should be made stronger and more stable to prevent the most common (rolling of the) ankle injuries. In almost every case I have witnessed, when the ankle of a walker or runner fails, it does so by rotating or turning to the inside, dropping the body outside and down. Sometimes the ankle gets torn up, sometimes the knee or shoulder takes the hit. Sometimes, you get lucky.

Grabbing the front half of the feet to facilitate this stretch is a good example of how the mechanics of a stretch, no matter how effective they may be for the targeted area, can simultaneously be detrimental to other parts of the body when one is not thinking things through.

Why do people grab their feet? It's the path of least resistance.

What can I say but, "Form, baby, Form!"

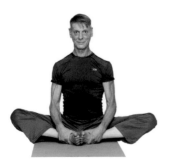

PHOTO 151

3. Lock your shoulders squarely into your trunk. Lift tall through the lower back and crown of the head to strongly align the back vertically over the hips. (As with the **Half Lotus Variation**, learning against a wall can be very helpful.)
    Once vertical, see how close you can pull the feet toward the hips—no rolling forward of the head and shoulders—and how wide you can open your knees.

Take a deep breath, lifting tall through the crown of the head. Feel the stability of those shoulders in lock down.

4. As you exhale, begin rolling the torso forward and down—starting from the top of the head. Keep your shoulders strongly in place.

    Pull with the arms, bending at the elbows as the torso lowers (Photo 152). When your forearms reach your thighs, press them into the thighs to open the thighs more as your body comes down.

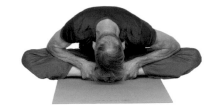

PHOTO 152

Nose to the toes, please. Belly freshly squeezing.

5. When you have reached the limits of what this position can do for you, slowly begin to straighten your knees (extend the legs along the floor—a few inches, pause, a few inches, pause—feet distancing from the hips).

    Nothing else changes. The legs remain rotated open, the body hangs forward. If you're tight, keep the hands attached to the ankles (or as low along the calf as flexibility permits), and continue to pull the body lower. If you feel loose here, you can let gravity and your legs do the work (Photo 153).

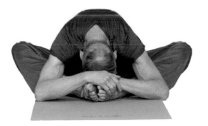

PHOTO 153

In either case, be sure to relax your neck and keep your belly engaged. A few inches, pause. A few inches, pause.

6. When you feel that your legs are as straight as they're going to go (still rotated open), grab your feet or your legs again and pull your body long (Photo 154), then point and flex the feet 8 to 12 times (Photo 154).

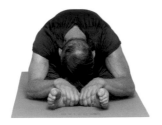

PHOTO 154

7. With the legs still as straight as possible, turn the knees in to their normal forward (upward) position and flex and point the feet 8 to 12 more times.

8. After this, keep the feet flexed, open the legs about 6 inches apart and, pulling (in good form) with the arms, try to bring your nose to the floor between your knees (Photo 155).

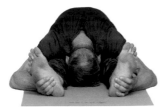

PHOTO 155

It's easy. It took me less than four years to accomplish, starting in my mid-twenties, working on it three or four times a day.

Of course, I needed that much stretch. You may not. Remember, flexibility is a property best tailored to the individual.

If this were my warm-up, at this point I would add some Crunches to really get the muscles warm. I would then proceed to **Pelvic Curls** and the **Working Supine Stretch** found in chapter II, then try to get some full Sit-ups in, before going on to **Leg Wide**.

LEGS WIDE

One often sees people begin this type of stretch by sitting on the floor, opening both legs wide and reaching, hanging or pulsing down the middle. If you're already quite warm, that might be acceptable.

I would argue, however, that you should always start to one side or the other, as stretching down the middle with both legs wide is the most stressful position possible for the inner thighs at this, their most delicate juncture (where they join with the hips).

One muscle in particular, the *gracilis*, is long, thin, and extends from the pubic bone, along the inner thigh, and its ligament crosses the knee to attach to the calf. When you stretch this long and thin muscle a little too much, it strains—or worse—very easily.

The pain of a strained *gracilis* is usually felt in the groin. Tends to last about three months. I'll leave the aching sensation to your imagination, unless you've already experienced the thrill.

For me, it's safer and more productive to begin with one leg wide at a time. Let's start there.

ONE LEG WIDE

1. Sit on the floor and open the left leg out to the side. Lift tall from the lower spine up and keep both hips firmly on the floor.
    Bend the right knee and open it to the side, drawing the sole of the right foot into contact with the left inner thigh (Photo 156). (It is important to bring the sole of the foot all the way into contact with the inner thigh.)

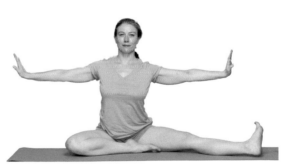

PHOTO 156

2. Place the right hand on the inside of the open right knee and press gently down. Reach out with the left hand to the left foot (or as far out the left leg as possible, with both hips remaining flat on the floor) and grab hold. Keep your shoulders in place.

3. Take a deep breath. Exhale and lower your body directly forward, between the hips (Photo 157), with the left arm pulling long and the bent right arm stabilizing through it's set shoulder and pressing hand.

The head and torso lay out and down over the middle of the hips.

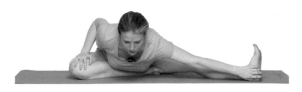

PHOTO 157

Though pulling with the left arm, do not take the body to the left; stay equidistant between the knees as you stretch and drop. The pull on the left leg is more to stretch that leg as the body travels down the middle of the hips and to supply, along with the right arm, stability during the exercise.

Avoid rolling the left knee forward. Try to keep it at least vertical, though, preferably, rotated open to the back.

4. When you reach your stretching limit, hold yourself there and try pointing and flexing the left foot a few times. Work all the way through the toes (Photo 158).

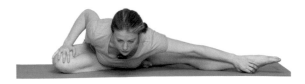

PHOTO 158

Don't forget to breathe.

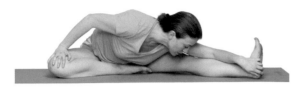

PHOTO 159

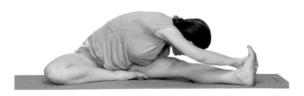

PHOTO 160

5. Continue pointing and flexing the left foot and draw your stretching torso—constantly at its farthest perimeter (supported by the arms)—in a semicircle around to the left, until the center of the chest is (roughly) aligned over the top of the leg (Photo 159).

6. Bring the right hand as far down toward the left heel as possible. If you can, reach across the left leg with the right hand and grab it from the outside (Photo 160).

The left hand presses down, back by the left hip, to stabilize and alter the angle of stretch. Place the heel of the hand and the inside of the wrist against your butt, and the fingers (splayed—for stability) reaching away from it. Continue stretching in this direction.

If you can't reach your foot, the fingers—of one or both hands—can reach under the bottom of the leg, which, when fully stretched, locks the fingers in place against the floor, assisting the grip.

Remember to keep your shoulders set, belly squeezing, and don't forget to breathe. Strong left knee, strong left foot and toes—pointed, flexed or performing both. Rotated open.

7. Take a deep breath. Exhale, release the hands, lift and rotate the torso—led by the right arm—to sit up and face front. Finish vertically aligned—shoulders squared—over the hips, torso facing forward. The arms reach out to the sides at shoulder height (Photo 161).

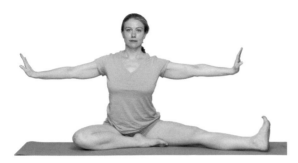

PHOTO 161

8. Flex the left foot, rotate the left leg open to the back and stretch it strongly, from the hip through the heel. Check that both hips are firmly grounded.
    Reach over the crown of your head (to the left) with the right arm (Photo 162). (Compare with the overhead ach in the Half Lotus Variation, step 7).

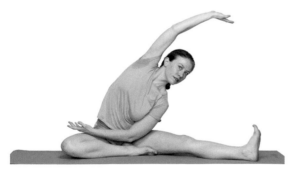

PHOTO 162

9. The left arm reaches down and across the lower belly (in front of the torso) to the right. Be sure to press your right elbow back above your head and turn both palms to the ceiling.

Simultaneously lean to the left as far as you can without rotating the torso (it continues to face front) or lifting the right hip (Photo 163).

The left arm reaching across the front of the belly helps to maintain the torso facing front, as it draws the left shoulder down and in toward the left hip.

This action also draws a stronger, more stable targeted stretch.

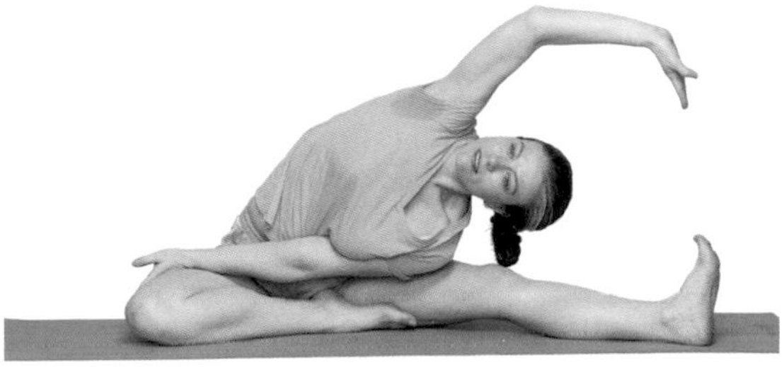

PHOTO 163

10. Using the right arm to lead, press it up and out to the right and down from the top of the shoulder, as you exhale and unbend to your vertical origin. Change your legs to the right side and repeat starting from step 2.

BOTH LEGS WIDE

As expressed previously, stretching, seated, with both legs wide, opens up an entire tender region of the body to great stress, which, if not properly managed, can engender moderate to merciless misery for a considerable amount of time. For this reason, I pause to remind you to always, when actively stretching in this position—whether static or fluid—use the strength of your belly, legs, feet and toes to assure the structural integrity of whatever strategy you may employ.

In passive mode, stretching is not as stressful, as gravity is the only force applied. Usually, good form and true relaxation will suffice to keep things safe.

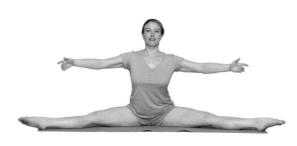

PHOTO 164

1. Begin sitting tall (if you need to, use a wall), both legs at their maximum safe width. Knees are strong and straight, either vertical or rotated open to the back (Photo 164). Feet and toes can be pointed or flexed.

   If this is new to you, definitely flex. Flexed feet in this position add inner thigh protection that pointed feet do not.

2. Rotate your torso to face the left leg. Place the right palm on the floor inside the thigh, and the left palm on the floor outside the thigh, at a moderate degree of stretch.

3. Reaffirm the right leg's stretch and the reach of its heel to the right, the foot's strong flex and the knee's outward rotation. Maintain the right hip firmly on the ground.

4. Inhale. Beginning with the head, exhale and roll the body down over the left thigh, with the intention of bringing the top of the head to the left knee.
   This is not a lengthening stretch in the normal sense. One should not try to reach out, stretching the back long toward the foot, but, rather, curl into oneself, toward the hip. A lifted spine and freshly squozen belly help considerably.

Be sure to roll down from the crown of the head. Avoid contracting the lower back (pulling it behind the hip) as you curl.

5. Stay there and inhale deeply. Exhale deeply. Though the belly is squeezing and the arms are providing support as needed, the back and spine should be relaxing more with every breath. You will feel the body rise with each inhale, and drop, incrementally, more with each exhale. Enjoy it.

6. When you're ready, roll your body back up, on the exhale, using your abs and lifting from the lower spine as you rise. Inhale as you face the right leg, and repeat.

7. Now go back to the left. Place the left hand on top of the left thigh and the right farther down the left leg, on top of the calf, if possible, about halfway to your full stretch.

As you exhale, take the chest toward the leg, reaching away from the hip (Photo 165). You're going for a medium stretch this time, prepping the targets (lower back and inner thighs) for the big one coming up.

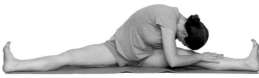

8. After going left, go to the right. Always keep the opposing leg stretching strongly to the opposing side and its hip firmly seated on the floor.

PHOTO 165

9. Now go for single-leg gold. From the starting position, place the left hand on the floor against the outside of the left hip, heel of the hand and inside of the wrist against the butt (this provides greater stability than reaching long with both hands). The right hand reaches long to grab the left calf or foot (Photo 166), the same hand positions as step 7 in **One Leg Wide**).

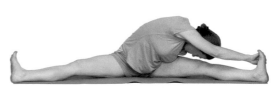

PHOTO 166

Take the body out and down and get that good stretch going. Once you're secure, you can reach out with the left hand as well, if you wish.

10. Now, the right side, if you please. Having achieved a good stretch in each of the legs individually, it is now much safer to go down the middle and work them both together.

11. Assume the starting position (Photo 167).

12. Here you have two options. You may roll forward and down from the crown of the head, or you can reach out long from the hips and lower back. The second is more stressful on the lower back, but it also offers more opportunity to open the hips (Photo 168)

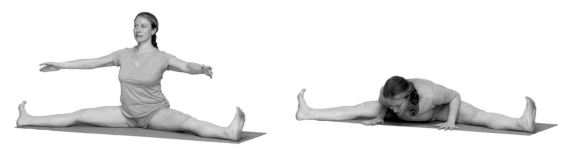

PHOTO 167   PHOTO 168

Whichever method you choose, use your hands on the floor in front of you, to control the weight of the body as long as needed. Once you are secure, you may reach wide to the calves or feet, or reach out, forward and long, as when the arms are extended on the floor and the body is forward and down in **Half Lotus Variation**, steps 5 through 7.

Strong feet, strong knees, strong butt, strong belly. When reaching with your arms, keep those shoulders down.

13. Once back in starting position, take the arms wide. Reach over the top of the head with the right arm, down and across the belly with left, and bend the torso to the left side, torso facing front as in steps 9 and 10, **One Leg Wide** (Photo 169).

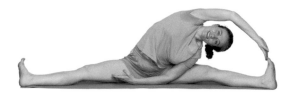

PHOTO 169

14. Go to the right. Repeat left and right four times. Use the muscles in your sides and belly to lift tall as you rise up and over the middle to the other side. Reach with those arms and press those shoulders down to strengthen the solid resolve in the torso. Rise on the inhale, bend on the exhale.

15. When you're ready to move on, put both hands on the floor, just behind their respective hips, and quickly pull your butt back, along the floor, and draw your legs together. It has been my experience that this "dismount" is far less painful than slowly pulling the legs in one at a time. Once they're together, shake them out. Bounce the knees lightly up and down a few times to restore comfort to the hips.

ON THE RECLINE

ALL O' YOUR TWIST

1. Lie flat on your back, arms wide on the floor, perpendicular to your body, in line with your shoulders, palms down. Knees bent vertically at just under 90 degrees (Photo 170).
Feet are together and pointed, with only the tips of the toes on the floor. (You'll be surprised what a difference this makes in your lower belly versus flat feet.)

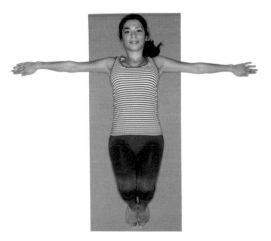

PHOTO 170

Inhaling, turn your head in one direction and your knees in the other.

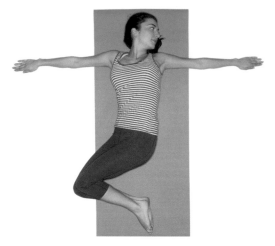

PHOTO 171

2. As you do so, reach out with the hand you are facing (opposing the knees) and secure your shoulder (Photo 171). The knees stay glued together, both for greater stretch and, together with a squeezing belly, greater stability in the twisting, arching torso. Holding the knees together in this manner will cause the upper foot to leave the ground. Keep it glued to the lower foot.

The strength in your inhale also helps to control the descent of the knees and the torque of the spine.

3. Exhale and squeeze your belly hard into the lifted side of your torso, from the ribs down into the hip. Use that squeeze to press your lifted hip into the floor. This will draw the knees up toward the other side from the belly, rather than from the thighs, and really work your waist. Press the lower back into the floor as the knees pass vertical alignment.
Don't forget to turn the head, in opposition, at the same time.

4. Inhale as the legs begin to drop to the other side. Control their descent. Reach away with the opposing arm once again. Repeat 20 to 30 times, and you'll get not only a great stretch, but a really good ab and trunk rotator workout—so long as you really work that squeezing exhale, contracting it into the lower back, and that expansive inhale, as the back arches, controlling and challenging the descent of the knees.

KNEES TO THE CHEST

1. Start reclining on the floor—knees bent vertically together, feet together and flat, arms by your sides. Roll up from your head and shoulders, bring your knees up slightly (lower back stays on the floor), and then reach as far down the calves as you can (preferably to the ankles), and wrap your arms tightly around your tightly bending legs, and pull your knees into your chest (Photo 172). Lock your arms together by gripping the back of one wrist with the opposite hand. Press your bending elbows into the legs and squeeze them together tightly (think arms as shrink wrap).

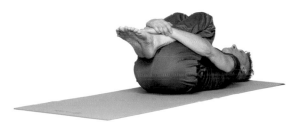

PHOTO 172

2. Using your arms only, pull your heels into your butt as close as possible, to extract the greatest bend from the knees.

Using the arms thusly relieves the legs of any working role in the stretch. Once shrink wrapped, they become dead weight, completely relaxed (the feet, too!), and are manipulated entirely by the strength and grip of the arms (and the lowering of the upper back and head to the ground). This dead weight approach allows a much freer stretch in the hips and lower back, our targets for the occasion.

Lock your shoulders down (and back, if they're rotated forward) and keep your upper back and head to—or near, it's a flexibility thing—the floor (long neck, please). This action will draw the lower back off the floor, or, at least, considerably increase your stretch.

The security of the grip directly impacts the safe support of the lower back in this stretch, as the arms are entirely responsible for controlling the load and not allowing it to rest on a lifted lower spine.

3. Try to pull the knees into the chest even further. Turn your head slightly to the left and take your legs slightly to the right (Photo 173).

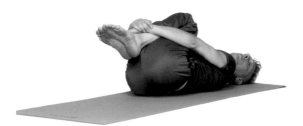

PHOTO 173

This brings the pressure of the floor to bear on one side of the mid to lower back, at roughly the level of the kidneys, pressing specifically into that area.

Proceed slowly and do not twist so far as to lose your balance. Breathe deeply and use your arms.

4. Exhale and rotate to the other side. You may hang out for a while on either side, alternate a couple of times, or work however you like. Once you assume the position, you'll know what to do.

Don't be surprised if one side reacts differently from the other. For the first two years I used this stretch, my left side felt fine and my right was ground zero for a vicious, aching pain, whose multitudinous fingers spread out in all directions across my back.

When using this stretch as part of your warm-up, I would suggest some leg lifts before going to the next stretch. If this part of your passive R&R, take it easy, to the extent that you wish, and save the leg lifting for another time.

RECLINING SINGLE-LEG STRETCH

1. Lie flat on your back, legs straight out on the floor.

2. Bend the left knee, lock your hands together around the front of it (at the top of the calf), and pull it into your (same side) shoulder, as far as you can (Photo 174).

    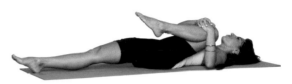

    PHOTO 174

    Allow the knee to turn out to the shoulder instead of driving directly into the chest. This will require a slight open rotation in the hip. Going directly into the chest with the knee puts the ribcage in the way of the stretching thigh, diminishing the opportunity (Photo 174).

3. Release the left hand and take hold of the bottom of your heel, the back of your heel or as far back up your calf as your flexible limit demands. Place the right hand on the back of the thigh and hold the thigh close to the

    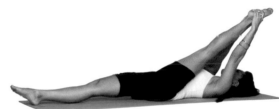

    PHOTO 175

    body as you point your left foot and try to extend the calf out over your head, using your left hand to pull against the stretch and help straighten the knee (Photo 175). For most of us the thigh will rise at least a little, if not a lot.

When the knee has straightened to the extent that the right hand is no longer helpful on the back of the thigh, add the left. Both now pull against the straightening knee, with the intent of bringing the top of the foot to the face.

Tight participants may need to hold the thigh, rather than the calf or foot, as they straighten the knee. The drawback is that pulling from the thigh, when trying to straighten the knee, imposes a natural propensity in the knee to bend. Pulling from the calf or heel, on the other hand, actually helps the knee to straighten, as it can press out against the pulling (in) of the hands.

4. Once a good, strong, stretch has been enjoyed, bend your knee back into your shoulder using your hands and arms.

5. Flex the foot strongly (Photo 176) and repeat steps 3 and 4.

You may perform this part of the stretch up to four times on each leg.

6. After this has been performed on each leg, repeat step 3, with either a pointed or flexed foot. Keep the stretching left leg straight and high.

7. Release the right hand and reach out wide to the floor on the right. Shoulder stable, palm down, flat on the floor.

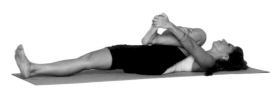

PHOTO 176

8. Take your stretched left leg—supported and guided by the left hand—open to the left side, as far as you can (Photo 177). Keep your body flat on the floor at all times (the reaching right arm helps).
    Once it's open all the way, release the left leg from the left hand (Photo 178) and stretch it out and down to join the right leg on the floor (Photo 179).

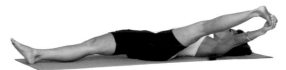

PHOTO 177

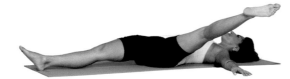

PHOTO 178

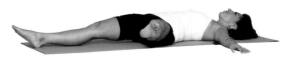

PHOTO 179

9. You guessed it—now do the right side!

WEATHER VANES

This is another stretch that one commonly sees in all exercising venues, though regularly done with little thought to technique, thus reducing benefits and increasing risks.

1. Recline—arms wide, palms down, legs long and together on the floor.

2. Reach out strongly with the left arm and secure the left shoulder to the floor. Bend the left knee vertically, lock the left foot behind the strongly stretched right knee, and then allow the left knee to drop to the right (Photo 180).

Keep the left leg anchored by the left foot behind that strong right knee.

Squeeze your belly (if you haven't already) and control the rise of your left hip. Keep your left shoulder down.

3. Turn your head to the left, and place your right hand on top of the left knee. You may press gently with the right hand, if you wish (Photo 181).

4. Breathe deeply. When you're ready, relax your body and release to the starting position.

5. Other side, please.

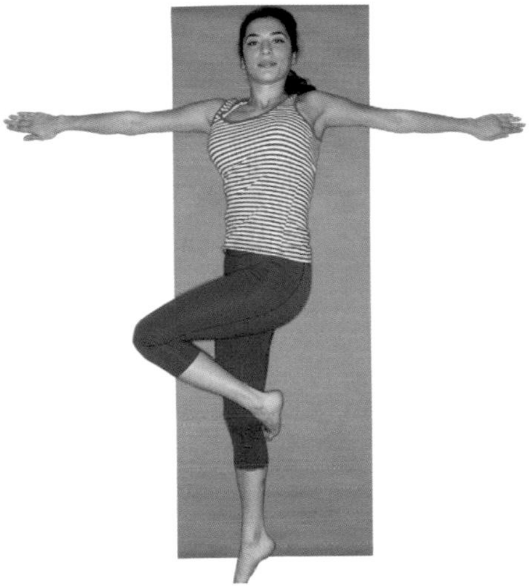

PHOTO 180

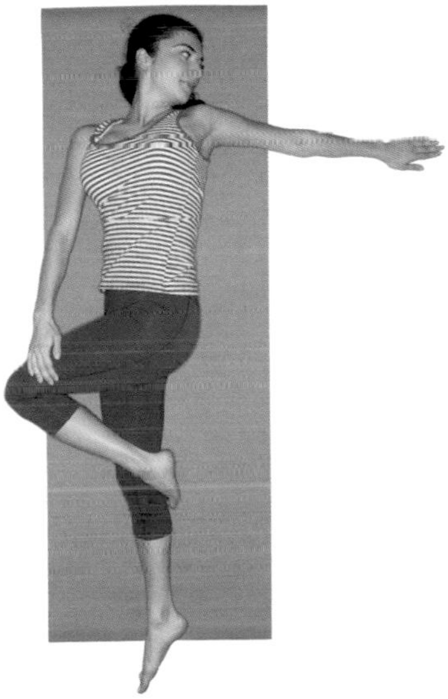

PHOTO 181

ON YOUR BELLY

THE COBRA

I include this traditional yoga form (an "asana") for two reasons: its widespread use and the almost consistently inadequate execution thereof.

Even with perfect execution, for many people (myself included), this stretch can be very tough on the lower back. Even for those who have no problem with it, there can be hidden, long-term ramifications, to continued misuse of this stretch, which may come calling—chronically—later in life. So, getting this right is really important

The problem is, for all the books in which I've seen this form explained (at present, a few dozen), and all the instructors I've heard instruct (perhaps a hundred), none have addressed the complete mechanical structure of the move. Some speak just to the visual basics, some add a few specifics, but few, if any, have even mentioned (and none completely) what I consider to be some critical points of interest—in the shoulders, the chest, the belly and the actual safest direction for the movement.

Here's my take on it. Shop and compare.

Let's review the objective: a well-supported, lifting arch of the upper body that lengthens and strengthens the back and spine while stretching the front of the torso and thighs.

Hmmm..."well supported"—better lock those shoulders down and squeeze that belly—"lengthen and strengthen the back and spine"—pushing straight up actually puts more crunch (weight and compression) in the back of the lower spine. Better to think forward and up, as though you were pulling the links of a chain out long as you lift them. This will require a slight forward change in the direction of your rise and a bit more effort (strengthening) in the shoulders, upper back and abs—"stretching the front of the torso and thighs"—once again, pushing straight up will not give all that forward and up will. Lead forward and up from the chin and chest—not lifting the chin will diminish the reach of the chest. Propel yourself by the (slow-motion) thrust of the arms.

O.K.

1. Lie flat on your belly, hands by (outside) your shoulders, palms on the floor. I usually face my fingers forward—it's easier to secure the shoulders, though some choose to turn the fingers in, which works more into the back of the upper arms (Photo 182).

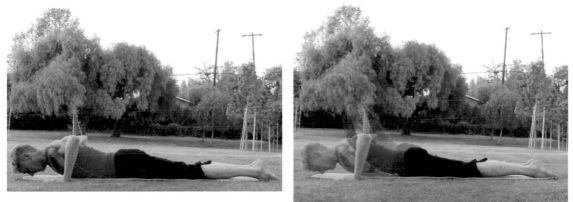

PHOTO 182

Legs are together. All is calm.

2. Let's start. Exhale. Press down and back with the shoulders. Inhale and steadily straighten the elbows (Photo 183). Belly squeezing all the way, press the chest forward and up, together with a rising chin.

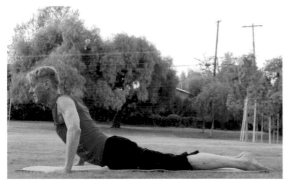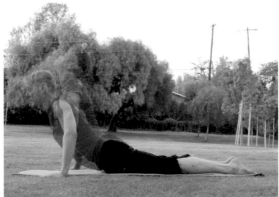

PHOTO 183

3. Rise as far as is comfortable. The legs remain long. You may leave them relaxed or, if you really want to work, squeeze your butt and stretch those limbs in the opposite direction of the rising chest and reach away through your pointing feet (Photo 184).

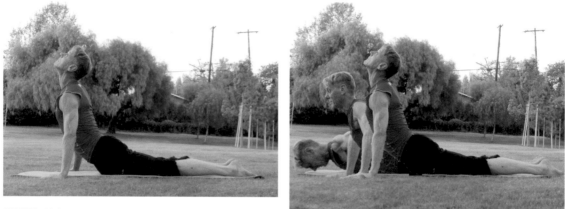

PHOTO 184

4. Once at your peak, do not relax into your skeleton and hold the position. Keep reaching for the stars. Take those shoulders farther down and back, making room for that thrusting chest leading the way to a higher tomorrow and squeezing your belly to support the spine.

5. You may lower as you exhale, or hang out up for a breath or two and then come down.

CAT CURL

If I use the **Cobra**, I'll want to combine it with a move to relieve the stress I have just placed on my poor lower spine. Another form from yoga, known as the **Cat Curl** or the **Child Pose**, is perfect in this role, and I am not alone in that belief.

To my understanding, any number of yogis and their followers, both famous and unknown, have regularly been attaching both posing children and curled kittens to the back ends of their cobra's for millennia.

For the purposes of this explanation, I'll go with **Cat Curl**.

1. You are prone, hands by your shoulders, the same starting position as for the Cobra (step 1) (Photo 185).

2. Inhale, press your torso up and back as you rise onto your hands and knees (Photo 186).

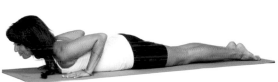

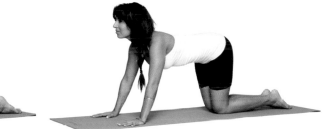

PHOTO 185

PHOTO 186

3. Exhale and contract (curl) your torso while taking your hips toward your heels (Photo 187).

Take your hips as far as they'll go. Leave your hands where they are. The arms will extend forward from the shoulders as the hips bend back.

4. Inhale. Now, there are two options. If you intend to return to **Cobra**, as you exhale, take your torso forward—elbows bending, snake low to the ground with that chest—and, as you stretch out, rise forward and up again.

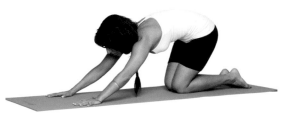

PHOTO 187

If you're ready to relax, as you exhale, take your arms wide and around, from the shoulders, along the floor to your feet. Turn your palms up, forget the world and focus on your breathing.

If you want more stretch in your hips in this pose, keep the feet together and open your knees. If it's in your back you want more stretch, keep those knees together.

5. I'm sure there is a limit on how long one should enjoy the **Cat Curl**, but I've never reached it. One teacher used to leave us in it for several minutes at the end of class, and I've done the same with my students.

It is very relaxing. Curl wisely, my friends.

However you stretch, whatever stretches you use—know what you're doing with every part of your body and why. Don't improve one thing at the expense of another.

If you don't stretch at all, you may as well go on to the next chapter, 'cause, sooner or later, I can almost guarantee you, you're going to need the information.

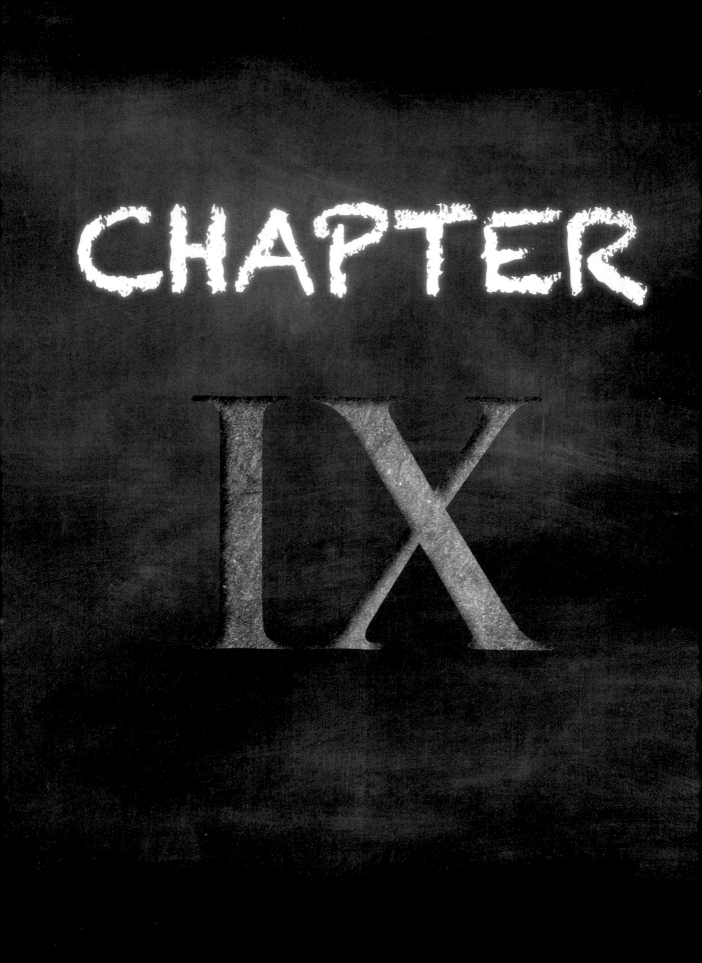

CHAPTER IX

CHAPTER IX: INJURY AND RECOVERY

As virtually every tunesmith has sung throughout the centuries, "Everybody hurts sometime." That's just the emotional truth of life (psychotics excepted). Split the first word in that phrase and you'll find the complimentary physical truth: Every **body** hurts sometime.

Perhaps you've heard someone claim that they've never been sick a day in their life. For their sake, I hope that's true. What I've never heard someone claim is that they've never been injured a day in their life.

The human body is far too complex a mechanism to function constantly and not have something go wrong from time to time. If we're lucky, most such anomalies—non-specific pinches, aches, pains—will take care of themselves and ease on out of our lives.

However, when they don't leave, when they nag a little louder each day, when they begin to wake you in the night, when you start to reorganize the way you live and move around them, it's time for a decision—do nothing and remain in lockdown, or find a way out.

Whether your injury is obvious from the instant it occurs, or whether it creeps up over the years to manifest some long uncared for mismanagement—unless surgery is the only option, there are recovery techniques that can help. Usually, when such injuries are sudden, and often with long-standing situations, a full return to healthy normalcy is possible.

Even with extenuating circumstances—a muscle in atrophy, slight joint deterioration, numbness in a certain position or, chronically, in an isolated area of the body—as long as it's safe to work on it, significant progress, in my experience, can be made. You may have to begin with very small, very slow, very careful movements, and it may be painful to try (sometimes it's actually relieving), but, with studied evaluation, a cautious strategy, patience and sincere dedication, you'll be surprised at how much you can improve.

If you don't think it's worth it, consider this: You can either spend some time in, what may be, a painful recovery and feel much better thereafter, or you can learn to live with it and spend the rest of your life in chronic pain or debilitation.

Personally, I'd go for that first one.

GETTING HURT

Of course, there are several things one can do to avoid getting hurt in the first place. Living life inside a healthy physical structure with healthful muscular support is most obvious, followed by not attempting things for which your body (strength, flexibility, skill) is not prepared.

Another important factor, often ignored, is hydration. A dehydrated body working out, or making a sudden, sharp movement, or even just holding a moderately stressful position, can easily come to harm. Muscles made of paste and glue might resist the job they are meant to do, leaving the only poetry in the motion an elegy to the sorrowful aftermath.

Last—and first—is diet. A body can't maintain, build or renew without the necessary nutrients.

Still, careful as we might be, even those most fit or skilled among us will fall prey to human frailty from time to time and suffer injury—though not necessarily from extreme pursuits. Our daily lives are full of physical challenges that go unnoticed, perhaps, due to their mundane nature, but are potentially injurious nevertheless. There's an old joke about the grace of dancers: They are beautiful onstage and hilarious off, famous for exiting the limelight in poised perfection, only to trip and take a nose-dive down the backstage stairs.

Turning the body, to one side or the other, when rising to one's feet (something we've all done mindlessly), can be fine a thousand times and drop you like a stone on the thousand and first. Getting out of the car, reaching back for that bag and giving it a tug (with a hyperextended shoulder and a twisting, rising lower back) has filled more than one person I've known with Delayed Onset Remorse. Even a slight misjudgment of a single step, a little tug on the arch of the foot that seems like nothing at the time, can leave you unable to walk the next morning.

WHAT CAN GET HURT

There are many dishes served at Injury's Bounteous Feast, and the doors are always open. How often have we found ourselves, unaware that we were even in attendance, supping from that table on a dish better left alone.

Injuries can be served on any part of the body, delivered to any particular muscle, tendon, ligament, joint or group of same, at the drop of a hat (literally!). Most come with a healthy portion of pain on the side.

Let us peruse the bill of fare.

1. **Muscles** can be pulled, strained, knotted and torn.

I differentiate "pull" from "strain" by the following: a pull is rather long, ropey and thickish; a strain is sharper, generally thinner in depth and burns more. Either of these may involve some degree of tearing.

A "knot" is felt as a lump of tightened muscle (fibers) interrupting the smooth normalcy of the muscle.

A serious tear is usually tender to the softest touch. Moving or supporting weight on the area is painful to impossible. It may bruise, swell and show symptoms from any of the previous three issues, which symptoms would tend to be more pronounced. Tears can be minor, involving only a small amount of the aggregate structural tissue (muscular, tendinous, ligamental, connective), or severe ("Cue the scream!").

2. **Tendons** can be strained and torn.

Tendons are not as full bodied as muscles and made from different tissue. Though they can strain fairly easily, I have rarely, if at all, found the term "pull" useful with tendons.

Tears can be minor (not uncommon) or major. Minors can usually be healed, fairly easily, with careful attention. Majors often require surgery.

3. **Ligaments** can be strained and torn.

Ligaments have little stretch capacity. Their job is to hold the joints securely together and, in some cases, cushion them. This creates a lower threshold for strain and tear.

4. **Joints** can be unevenly or overcompressed, overstretched or dislocated. Unless the bone is broken, the resulting injuries are purely cartilaginous, ligamental, tendinous and neural in composition.

5. **Nerves** can be pinched, compressed or otherwise pressured by any of 1 to 4 above, creating a painful response anywhere along the line of the nerve, not necessarily where the problem lies.

In addition, nerves can be so damaged that the signals sent along them do not reach, or fully reach, some or all of the muscles they govern. This can result in numbness and a partial or complete failure of the muscles to perform, inhibiting one's ability to move the affected part of the body normally. If the injury remains unaddressed, the muscles will begin to atrophy, which is to say, waste away and decrease in size.

I have had three such injuries that were serious, and I recovered from them all. One in my left calf, one in my right thigh and one, as collateral damage from a neck injury, that deadened the left side of my upper lip and part of my cheek.

Thankfully, I got past the facial infirmity quickly. Several times a day, when alone, I would work through various expressions and movements that invited the numbed area to participate. Within three weeks, I was eating and drinking again without worrying about spillage—smiling and laughing again with my countenance intact.

The other two took considerably longer. Completely unresponsive for quite some time, in both cases the numbed muscles shrunk dramatically, and there were times I thought I was stuck with a permanent loss of movement. (The left calf affected both my ability to rise onto my toes [i.e., releve, tiptoe] and stabilize there. The right thigh was in one of my quads, the one that drives my leg up when it is rotated open and to the side at 45 degrees.)

However, I never gave up. I continually challenged the numbed muscles on a daily basis to do their job. Eventually, they woke up, got back to work full-time, and regained full strength. It took over a year for the left calf and a full year and a half for the right thigh.

From these, I learned one more lesson in patience and perseverance.

RECIPES FOR DISASTER

As I mentioned, all one has to do to injure oneself is stay alive. Yet such a simple phrase can hardly suggest the myriad possibilities available for the corporeal human to come to harm.

1. **Impact** (into the ground when running, stepping, climbing stairs; on a heavy bag or against focus mitts when punching or kicking; getting knocked down, thrown down, etc.)

One's alignment can be perfect, yet too much force against too strong a resistance can overload the body's ability to safely absorb the shock. With poorer form, any number of body parts can suffer very easily. The weakest link (in support and alignment) will be the first to fail, yet it may not be the last.

Impact injuries can include joint compression and various strains, tears (including tears of the connective tissue that holds muscles against the bones, as with shin splints) and pulls (which may soon knot up), as well as bruising and swelling. In severe cases, impact can cause stress fractures (at extremes, even clean breaks) in the bones themselves.

2. **Repetitive stress** (too much of a good thing)

Repeating the same action over and over, whether through formal exercise over a shorter period of time, or through poor postural habits continued for decades, can overstress muscles, joints and nerves. Too much running, too much pumping, too much sleeping always on the same side can wreak various havocs on your physical composition.

It might creep up when you're resting, a pulsing line of pain in one specific area of a muscle or joint, that slowly increases over time and with certain movements. It may happen suddenly, as with a cramp, pull, strain or tear in a muscle or ligament overworked from too many exercised reps (dehydration can play a role here).

When repetition combines with impact, we often feel the anomaly begin in one misaligned rep (or step). Too often in such cases, the sharp, immediate pain goes away with corrected form, and we push on through the work, not realizing that the damage is already done. But when the adrenaline stops pumping, the pain comes a-thumping. Later that night, or next morning, we find that out.

Repetitive stress can affect huge portions of one's musculoskeletal system. With the exception of specific injuries to the belly of a muscle, in many cases I've dealt with, though the injury occurs in only one area, pain appears in numerous spots along the associated neural pathways, often a good distance away.

For instance, with a common type of shoulder repetitive stress, though the injury will be rooted in the area of the shoulder blade, upper back or neck, the roots of the problem are never felt. The initial pain appears across the front of the shoulder.

And, often, with this type of injury, the pain extends down the arm, even through the wrist and into the hand and fingers. Yet, though one can find associated and treatable irregularities in various muscles throughout the line of pain, until the roots are addressed—and the mechanical causes of the stress are corrected—you're just treating the symptoms, not reaching for the cure.

How to figure what's what with repetitive stress and get beyond it is made clear in chapter X, **Recovery Techniques**.

3. **Range of Motion**

One may destroy all good things by overchallenging one's ROM.

Whether through the rapid exuberance of uncontrolled swings, arches and twists, or from trying to support or move too much force at the extended end of one's muscular reach (in the breadth of **Chest Flies**, for instance, when the weights at the ends of the levers—in this case, the arms—dangerously overload the fulcrums of the movement—the chest and shoulders—at their moment of widest stretch and highest physical stress), ROM injuries can be very painful and regularly take some weeks to recover.

At the easier end, you get pulls and strains of muscles, tendons and ligaments. At the tougher end, you face issues that may encompass seriously tearing these, as well as overcompression and hyperextension of the joints, and undue wearing and even tearing of the cushioning cartilage between and inside the joints, which are essential to viable movement.

Protecting ROM does not only mean keeping movement within safe boundaries. It also means developing a thorough understanding of how much resistance your body (or its parts) can safely handle, in any given position, within those boundaries. Actively using the muscles, through every motion to control all aspects of the movement, is essential.

I've seen too many hips, shoulders and spines injured when thrown too freely through the air, too many elbows, knees and hips injured when punching and kicking the air with poor technique, to think that anyone's body automatically knows the right thing to do. Training is essential.

Similar problems arise in yoga, Pilates and the like, when challenging ROM positions, requiring strong support throughout the body, and thoughtful alignment are left wanting.

1. Hyperextension

When a joint is bent in a direction contrary to that in which it was intended to move, or, in the case of the ball and socket, when it is forced open farther than the structure will safely allow, hyperextension is the name of the game. A common example is found among those whose joints, for various reasons, are a bit looser naturally (though often called "double-jointed", the expression is inaccurate), allowing their knees and elbows to bend somewhat in the opposite direction of their normal function (such people must be particularly careful to prevent damaging these joints).

Many ROM injuries result from thoughtless Hyperextension. A good awareness of—and control over—the movements for which the different joints are intended is essential.

5. Resistance overload

The healthful side of this phrase is incumbent to weight training—one overloads the muscles with heavy resistance. Done right and regularly, this makes them grow in size, strength, and wisdom.

Overload them too much, too frequently, or with too poor form however, and rip!—crunch!—tear! Drop those weights and order some caviar, 'cause your muscles are toast.

Of course, resistance overload injuries can happen in any number of other ways outside the realm of formal exercise in daily life (push that car, lift that couch). In heavy situations, think before you act.

6. **Changing speed and dynamics**

An easy injury to come by is a pull, strain or tear when training, at length, with mixed speed and dynamics. An arm reaching works differently from an arm punching; a smooth rhythm works differently from a sharp rhytm; and changing from one to the other can sometimes spell trouble, particularly for a body that, for whatever reason, is not prepared. I've seen this type of injury especially in track and field, martial arts, dance and gymnastics.

Muscles inadequately trained, inadequately warmed-up, dehydrated or overworked often respond poorly when the game is changed. Muscles driven steadily at one rhythm and one intensity may find switching to another too radical a task.

Consider the difference between endurance running and sprinting. Working continuously at a strong but (relatively) moderate pace—as in an endurance run—the leg muscles engage in a rhythm of contraction and release that is smooth and even, and a dynamic force (intensity of landing, pushing off) that is fairly modest. Though they grow tired, once used to this, the legs can continue for quite some time.

However, if after a good endurance run, you change to sprinting, a new rhythm and dynamic range are introduced. Sprinting requires maximum power, rapid-fire contractions and push-offs and faster, longer-reaching forward strides, as hard as you can for short bursts of time.

Legs worn down by long endurance can have a hard time with the stability, speed and timing of rapid contraction and release. The greater demands of sprinting can cause muscles to "lock" or "freeze up" in the middle of a fast contraction (overcontracting), or a fast release (by refusing to stretch out when called upon). This can cause either searing pain (a strain or tear) or, in the case of a knot or pull, one of two options: the feeling that one has just been whacked, in one specific area, with a baseball bat, or an unrelenting sense that some hellish demon has reached inside your body and is squeezing it for all it's worth.

If this happens in one of your legs when you're sprinting, you may rely on the ground rising rapidly to your cheek, your hands grasping furiously to the pain, your torso contorting, your face distorting, and an anguished cry rising that you soon realize is your own. Oh, and a four- to six-week journey to relative recovery (unless you're **really** hurt).

Similarly, with the shoulders, arms and torso—in fact, any part of the body—too many changing dynamic challenges to a muscle (or group of same) or too much dynamic repetitive motion, can reap the same rewards described for the legs previously. Slow and fast punches, Crunches, kicks, reps with weights, even just reaching rapidly up and down in the air, when muscles are overtired, can bring a big freeze the moment you pour on the speed.

(If this sort of injury is to your taste, and you don't want to bother with wearing the muscles out before you can hurt yourself, simply skip your warm-up and jump right into a hard workout cold. You can achieve much the same result.)

Any of the injuries mentioned may occur singly or in combination. The choice is seldom ours to make. Once injured, however, the next move is entirely up to us.

GETTING INVOLVED

SEEKING PROFESSIONAL HELP

Once an injury has occurred, it needs to be taken care of. Let me say straight off the bat, if you feel you should see a doctor, do so. You may need to. Even if it turns out you don't, a doctor's opinion can prove beneficial. Though it's been my experience that doctors who regularly exercise themselves have a greater understanding of exercise related injuries than those who don't, whether the advice received turns out to be helpful or not, whether the diagnosis is good or bad, there is always something to learn from a competent professional's perspective.

What I don't recommend is blindly following a professional's advice. Get involved. Knowledge is power. If you don't fully understand the reasons and methods of what you're being told, ask for more explanation. Improve your understanding. Become better equipped to recognize what works for you and what doesn't, what will heal you more rapidly and more completely. The more you know the whys and hows of doing what you're doing, the better you'll get it done.

Perhaps it's just a natural curiosity in my character, but I always want to know why what's being done to me, or recommended to do, is appropriate and best for the situation at hand. After all, I'm the one who has to live with the outcome.

My own experiences with physical therapists, chiropractors, massage therapists and acupuncturists has been limited and mixed. Though I believe all of these approaches have intrinsic value, in each you will find practitioners both great and not so great. As in any walk of life, ability varies with each individual. Still, any professional will have a better chance to help you if he or she is well experienced in relation to your problem.

Paradoxically, experience can also be misleading. As I've said, not all bodies are the same, and similar symptoms in two different people might require two separate solutions. In a more experienced caregiver, it might be easy to assume that the fiftieth person with that kind of pain in that spot will be healed using the same techniques as the previous forty-nine, and therefore confidently fail to examine the patient as thoroughly as necessary to discover the complete truth.

Sometimes the unexpected becomes the overlooked.

PHYSICAL THERAPISTS

I've only seen a few physical therapists myself, in New York in my twenties, when my lower back first threatened my ability to continue dance training. They were in residence at a professional sports clinic at a prestigious New York hospital. Though they were fairly quick to define my problem (the genetic hairline fracture mentioned earlier in this book), I was a rare case, they told me, the first they'd ever seen in person, and they weren't quite sure what to do.

They researched all the available pertinent material, did their best to assess the situation and eventually suggested spinal fusion surgery.

Not wanting to give up any of my hard won range of motion and mobility without a fight, I asked for any alternative. They said it was unknown territory, but gave me their best guesses for therapy, a series of passive stretches to be done two or three times daily. For the next few weeks, I followed their instructions with sincere intent, but it only made things worse.

I felt, or sensed, that passive, static stretches were not the key. But, what was? I decided that, if there were solutions to be found, they were mine to find. I would have to begin searching for answers on my own.

However, the doctors did give me one very good piece of advice, which I have kept close in mind ever since. "With your condition," I was told, "you'd better exercise every single day of your life or never at all."

I immediately mistrusted that "never at all" part, and have since discovered that "every single day" is a bit more pointed than my actual truth. Which is good, for, currently, I rarely get in seven days of exercise per week. On really good weeks I'll hit seven, but my average is more like five. I've found I can maintain my spinal health with as few as three workouts per week, but only for a limited time (three weeks tops). Any less than that—or if I hit one of those rare occasions when I miss a week or 10 days—and the security of my lower spine is compromised. One wrong move—and I never know what that move will be—could drop me in a heartbeat and keep me down for weeks.

As for secondhand accounts of physical therapists, I have heard many, and they also break between excellent and poor results. Once again, the best seem to have physically learned their stuff in an up close and personal way, along with their academic study.

I applaud this approach. To my mind, until you gain understanding in your own body through your own physical training, your education in exercise related matters will be wanting.

CHIROPRACTORS

The best chiropractor I ever saw (and the only one I saw more than once) had spent years administering to a prominent ballet company. He was a traditional chiropractor, what some refer to as a "bone-popper" or "bone crusher," and he didn't believe in stringing people along. His philosophy was simple: "Come to me when you have a problem; don't get hooked on regular visits."

Personally, his methods gave me, and many other performers I knew, great relief. You saw him, he fixed you if he could (every time but one for me, when my genetic spinal infirmity had reared its ugly head) and you got on with your life. I never met anyone who had been to him who did not praise him to the skies.

The worst fixable injury I had, when I relied on his abilities, was a painful compression at the base of my neck. I waited a year before I went to him, trying to fix it on my own, but I could neither restore full mobility nor relieve the bulk of the pain.

So I went to Louis, but I didn't mention my problem. (I never told him what was wrong when I went to him, as sort of as a test, I guess, to see if he would figure it out.)

The man had a gift. Every time I saw him, as he worked through my joints, he would identify the anomaly the moment he approached it. Always blew my mind.

The same was true on this visit. He spotted the trouble immediately. After giving the rest of my skeleton a good working over, he firmly gripped my head, lengthened the stretch through the back of my neck, and gave it a good, sharp pull out from my shoulders.

It was a nice try, but nothing changed. He suggested we wait a week and try again.

Actually, I had to go twice more. The second visit went much as the first but, on the third visit, when he pulled my neck out sharply, a loud pop came from the base.

My mobility improved almost immediately. The muscles in the area were pretty sore for three or four days, and then my neck was right as rain. That particular injury has never bothered me again.

Though he was the only chiropractor I ever used who really impressed me, I have no doubt there are some excellent ones out there. Chiropractors can be very helpful, depending on the type of injury.

MASSAGE THERAPISTS

As for professional massage, I think it's more of a personal preference thing. There are so many styles, so many schools of thought, it seems to really come down to what you like and what's effective. Of course, the skill level of the individual therapist will certainly influence the work, whatever style is employed.

I have enjoyed Swedish massage, Japanese Reiki, acupressure, and, happily, during my dance years, the occasional set of skilled fingers attached to one lovely colleague or another. Though the latter was more intriguing, in terms of strict massage, acupressure heals the body best, in my experience.

The only thing I would add is to be careful who you let manipulate your body. Sometimes, if you don't feel something the way a therapist thinks you ought to, they may knead you too hard, twist you too far, dig that knuckle in, or otherwise overstress your body in ways that leave you less than thrilled, much less relaxed or comfortable.

This has happened a few times to me. My last incident was with a massage therapist of several years experience.

Knowing I was flexibly educated, this person wanted to show me a twisting release (stretch) he liked for the hips and trunk, sort of showing off to me, I guess, something he thought was new. Though I was hesitant to let another person demonstrate a push and pull technique on me, he was a colleague and, not wishing to offend him, I agreed.

However, I'd been working my flexibility for more than 20 years at the time, and, when I was manipulated into that position, I didn't feel anything special. This seemed to frustrate my colleague, who then proceeded, despite my words of caution, to pull a bit too hard, push a bit too hard, and, ultimately, overtwist my spine.

I felt the sharp stab of pain, the lightning-fast freeze and release of my abs in response, the snowballing inevitability that my midsection would soon grip into an immovable mass of searing unhappiness. But I had years of practice masking the symptoms of a back in chaos, and I didn't want my colleague to feel guilty.

I managed to get to my feet looking pretty normal, and I left the gym minutes later, before I quit looking so. Driving home, I had to roll onto my side in the driver's seat, to be able to apply pressure to the brakes with my left foot. Once home, I immediately collapsed.

For the next four days, sitting, standing or walking were major accomplishments. At night, I slept very little, having to lay flat on my upper back, while supporting, with pillows, a full twist in my waist and hips, thereby lying on my side from the hips down. It was the least painful position I could find, but that's not saying much. I ached powerfully and consistently. Beginning my rehab, two days later, was no fun either.

I no longer allow others to manipulate my structure, unless I know them very well, or they come highly recommended from someone in whose opinion I trust.

ACUPUNCTURE

My experience with acupuncturists is almost entirely second hand, and it's usually in the form of praise for one particular acupuncturist. First hand, I have seen only one. Two sessions were given me as a Christmas gift, and I decided to use them to see if acupuncture could help relieve the restless leg syndrome that had been growing in me, slowly, for years.

On my first visit, the needles were placed traditionally, where the doctor thought their input would best relieve the disruptive neural signals causing the sensations, not at the origins, as I sensed them, of the sensations themselves. Unfortunately, over the next few days, nothing changed, good or bad.

A couple of weeks later, I went again. I hoped, as RLS was still fairly unheard of, and the acupuncturist in question had never treated anyone for it before me, he wouldn't be offended if I asked him to try the placing the needles in places I suggested.

He was fine with the idea, so I asked him to place them in the areas I felt were the origins of the aberrant neural signals. I'm happy to say the treatment had good success. I was not completely relieved but, for the next three months or so, the symptoms were both less frequent and less severe. (Had I had the money, at the time, to continue seeing him, I would've continued the experiment to see how far I could heal.)

Do not think, from this anecdote, however, that I am implying I somehow understood acupuncture better than this trained professional. Not at all! All I suggest is that my years of physically suffering from a growing problem with RLS, and an intimate knowledge of those parts of me that had been repeatedly injured, had, in this case, perhaps given me a better understanding of where the problem lay, as it related to my body, than the understanding the acupuncturist gained from his initial examination.

Though professionals study long and hard to master their areas of expertise, no one is all knowing or infallible. If you don't feel you fully agree with the answers you're getting, or the prescribed therapies are coming up short, get yourself more involved. Get a second opinion, talk to your friends, read magazines, books on the subject, or look up your problem on a medical website. See what you can learn for (and about) yourself.

DETERMINING THE SOURCE OF AN INJURY

Unless surgery is necessary, there is quite a bit you can do on your own to determine the origin, nature and possible paths to recovery of an injury. Considering it's your body, it only makes sense to learn as much about its healthful recovery as you can.

Two things you don't want to do when trying to assess how you've hurt yourself are to cause more injury and cause more pain. So, please, if you must err during your examination, do so on the side of caution.

Injuries felt the moment they happen, tend to be more severe than injuries that come on gradually. The injured area tends to be more (very) sensitive to touch, more limited in function and require a longer period of recovery.

Injuries that come on slowly are usually dealt with more easily, provided they are attended to when they first make them selves known. Left unaddressed, they often worsen over time, become chronic and require a period of recovery lengthened in relative proportion to the length of the delay you took before doing anything about it.

Especially when an injury worsens over time, the pain may be felt in one place though the problem actually originates in another. Some long-term injuries have, or can develop, multiple sources of damage, weakness and misalignment. Even immediate injuries can have collateral damage to related systems that remain unrecognized until more damage has been done. It is even possible to fail to recognize the primary source of an injury—at all—at first, which almost certainly extends the time necessary for recovery.

For all these reasons, it pays to first approach any injury with a calm and even perspective. No matter how much it hurts, a relaxed mental and emotional state is primary, not only to mitigating the immediate pain and any tenderness felt thereafter, but also to doing things right and doing them best. Heightened emotions, a mind focused acutely on the pain; fear, anxiety, anger, all make the senses—and muscles!—freeze up.

If you feel the injury is bad, you may want to wait 24 to 72 hours (or even longer) before approaching anything, other than home, or a doctor, rest and relief. If, on the other hand, you're ready to proceed, do so with calm, even breathing, a clear mind and a gentle hand.

Different kinds of injuries, different parts of the body, differing sensations of pain and differing visible symptoms will require different approaches, both to figuring out what's wrong and how to fix it.

For instance, a joint injury obviously caused from a sudden, overstressed misalignment—such as rolling the ankle—which results in throbbing, possibly sharp pain, tenderness and stiffness in movement, visible inflammation and probably bruising, gives you a good idea, from the beginning, how to approach the problem. (If you have to stay on it, tape the ankle before it swells too much. Later, at home, apply acupressure to the top of the calf at the back and sides of the knee. Work evenly across and down through the muscles, until you find those lovely points of painful release. Then press and hold. Below the ankle, do the same outward through the toes, especially through the arch and the top of the foot. **Do not** get closer to the injured ankle than feels safe.)

In a different joint injury scenario, however, there could be no immediate cause, no inflammation or stiffness, no visible signs, just a curious pain that slowly has grown, over days and weeks, in certain positions or movements, or when the body has been left in a default position for lengths of time. This problem is not so clear.

It could have several causes. The joint could be repetitively misaligning, overcompressing or overstretching when in use and under duress. It could be a strained tendon, aching where it crosses the joint. It could be a ligament. The pain could be caused from some distance, a signal telegraphed along a neural system being stressed by a muscular imbalance farther away, such muscles also usually found to have been habitually placed in the same situation day after day, as when always sleeping on the same side, always carrying with that arm, always allowing your knees to roll in or out, either standing or seated. Any of these can be symptomatic of "Repetitive Stress Syndrome," in which both alignment and usage issues must be addressed.

Particularly, though not exclusively, joint pain in an older adult, with probable stiffness and possible inflammation, could be exacerbated by arthritis.

In approaching injury assessment, develop a vocabulary that makes sense to you. Think of adjectives to describe your pain. Be precise. With so many symptoms out there, each serving as an indicator of the type of injury sustained, clarity is essential. If you're assisting another's injury, ask them what it feels like before you start.

I find descriptors such as burn(ing), rope(y), thick, knotted, loose, tight, heavy, numb, stiff, aching, electric, wiry, fluttering and sharp to be common and useful choices.

THE ROLE OF ACUPRESSURE

A great way to assess, and begin to recover from, an injury, is to use acupressure and its associated techniques. Acupressure is the application of intense, steady, unmoving pressure in one spot to release, relieve and relax any knotted, stressed or frozen soft tissues.

My tools of choice are fingertips and tennis balls. The fingertips are powered by internal strength, tennis balls do best when gravity supplies the pressure. Both are small enough to be precise, and soft enough, when used reasonably, to do no harm. (See chapter X, Recovery Techniques, The Pain of Recovery.)

These techniques have saved my backside, and the backsides of some of my clients, students, neighbors and friends, more than once, and are, to my mind, indispensable. I have more than two decades of experience with acupressure now and am continually amazed at its ability to help the healing process and rapidly diminish pain.

However, before you can jump in with hard pressure on one right spot, you've got to know the terrain. You've got to figure out what's going on before you can try to fix it.

When using fingertips, first press smoothly and gently, with the fingertips together, along the lines and breadth of the muscles that are in the line of pain, to define the length and breadth of the injury. (Begin from well outside the injured area and work your way in slowly.) Then, use the fingertips to drum, as though on a tabletop, or rub gently in a small, circular motion, along the muscles, to find what's sore and to begin the softening of any over-tight muscles and tendons. You may work toward the pain or away from the pain.

Once you have a good idea of where the problems lie, apply acupressure—start gently—as necessary. There are usually a few specific spots that beg for more attention when pressed upon. Give as they require. Work every place that feels good to work. Such places are the keys to success. (For an example of these techniques in a specific situation, see chapter X, **What to Do** from **The Neck and Shoulders**).

If the pain is not that strong to begin with, or a fairly recent development, you may feel relief even as you continue to apply pressure, or shortly after you stop, and that may be the end of it. The pain may not return.

In a more serious or chronic situation, you may feel a bit more sore, after you stop, and relief may not come until the next day. As well, the pain will most likely return and have to be treated regularly, with these same techniques, for some time. Failure to do so, especially in severe cases, may cause a reversal of fortune.

I once worked on a woman with extreme plantar fasceitis in her left heel (see chapter X, **Calves and Ankles**). Very painful, left untreated for years, when I met her she rarely walked, leaned heavily on a cane or crutches when she did, and relied, usually, on a wheelchair.

She had allowed no one but doctors and therapists to touch her below the knee, though their efforts to heal her had been unproductive. After speaking with her about her condition, she hesitatingly agreed to let me see what I could do.

I began, very gently, well away from her heel, all the way up into the back of her knee. I asked and was told that none of the professionals she had seen had addressed this area.

(I figured they'd never had plantar fasceitis. Well, I had—Big Time! And I'd had to keep running every day, mile after mile, leading my boot camp, over the pavement and rough terrain of the foothills. I had to learn real quickly what was going on or chop off my foot and glue on a peg.)

I worked the top of the woman's calf. I soon found the right spot, and, when I applied pressure, she felt the painful relief (pain of recovery) all the way down into her injured heel. She let me continue, and I very slowly worked down the line of her pain, into the meat of her calf muscles.

From there, I spent a full hour making my way, ever so slowly, down into her heel and out through the bottom of her foot. Once I reached the ends of her toes, I finished.

I was sure I had done her some good, but I was surprised as hell when she exclaimed that she felt almost pain free. She stood up, moved around the room and exclaimed that she could walk, freely and comfortably, for the first time in years.

I was happy for her, but I knew what was coming. I told her that, after so long an infirmity, this new freedom was purely temporary. I assured her that, in a few hours, the pain and tightness would return, most likely with a vengeance, the affected muscles angry at having been awakened after so many years of tormented sleep.

I suggested either she, or her boyfriend, who had observed my work with close attention, massage her calf out again at that time, and every time, probably a few times a day, over the next few weeks, if she was to gain any lasting recovery. She didn't seem thrilled at the prospect, and I feared she would not do it.

Sad to say, her pain did return, and vengefully. She again wouldn't let anyone touch her, she didn't do the work herself, and was soon back where she began. As I understand it, she chose to rely on medical solutions and now uses electrical stimulators, implanted down the backs of her legs, to mitigate the pain and help her to walk.

To my mind, this woman was lucky and didn't appreciate it. Her severe symptoms were caused by something that could easily be fixed, that had just gotten ridiculously out of hand. Most people with such symptoms remain infirm with no complete solution at all, much less an easy one that is, literally, at their fingertips.

I know it's scary, sometimes, going into new territory, especially when pain is involved. But, when it's just fingertips and tennis balls, and you can start as gently as you wish and as far from the injury as you like, it's not that threatening a prospect. Try it out. The pain you save may be your own.

INFLAMMATION AND BRUISING

Inflammation and bruising bear a thoughtful eye when detecting the type and degree of an injury. That either occurs at all is already an indicator of degree, though either can sometimes make things look much worse that they are.

Almost always found immediately at the sight of an injury, neither necessarily occurs on the injury itself. I have seen inflammation and swelling on the inner side of my ankle, while the debilitation (of stability, control and support) and primary pain occurred on the outside, with no visible swelling.

Either may be found on, above, below and opposite the injury (for instance, a top of the wrist injury that causes bruising or inflammation on the underside of the wrist as well) and may remain for some time after the injury has otherwise apparently healed.

A degree of inflammation is usually a good thing, beneficial in cushioning and protecting an injured area from further trauma. Too much, however, is too much, and ice and elevation may be needed to bring it down. Bruising can show up either rapidly or slowly, within minutes or overnight. I don't know that bruising is of any positive value after an injury, other than as an indicator, in this case, of the healing process.

Though acupressure will do you no good at the site of inflammation and bruising—applying pressure too close to either of these will cause unnecessary pain and, possibly, prolong your punishing predicament—you can, quite beneficially, work in the neighborhood.

Work well away from the sight, on muscles that might affect the area. Along with pinpoint pressure, smooth, strong rubbing along the muscles—always in the direction away from the injury, can be very helpful.

In some situations, bruising and inflammation become mobile. Under the influence of Earth's gravity, and centrifugal force, if the site is in the arms and legs, either or both can travel downward through the body. An impact above the eye might inflame and bruise below it. A hard impact to the upper thigh could send the initial inflammation and bruising on a week long, scenic tour down to the ankle.

Pain, thank goodness, is not a guaranteed traveling companion in such cases, but, if it hooks a ride, watch out. Apply the same acupressure approach mentioned above to soften the torment.

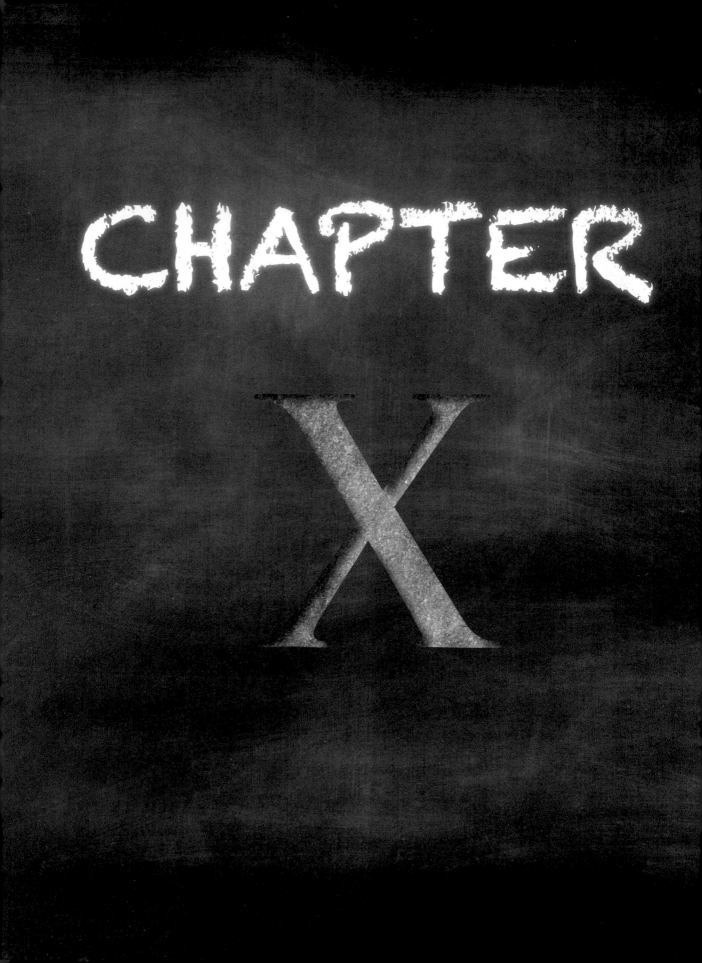

CHAPTER

X

CHAPTER X: RECOVERY TECHNIQUES

Immediate injuries require immediate attention, and the approaches are pretty obvious—assess the damage, assure that no more damage is done, and do what can be done to relieve the pain and aid recovery. If there are significant sympathetic injuries in other parts of the body, they'll probably show up when you start to move, as when getting back on your feet, bending over or reaching.

Chronic injuries, on the other hand, and injuries that appear the next morning, or more slowly over time, often have origins that are less obvious or more complex. The sight of the pain may be merely the symptom, not the problem itself. In such cases, in my experience, recovery efforts made at the sight of the pain often have little or limited effect. The root causes must be identified. This may require time, patience, calm, clear thought, a gentle touch and, when appropriate, movement begun slowly and gently.

A big factor in recovery, either immediate or long-term, will be the mental and emotional state of the injured. The scare of severe pain, the fear of the unknown, the perceived ramifications of a disrupted daily routine, all bring tension and stress to a body that really needs to relax.

So, once something has happened, it's happened. Collect yourself and deal with it. However bad the injury may be, calm is your friend. Deep, relaxed breathing is your friend. Clarity is your friend. These will help you determine what action is necessary. Panic just grips the body and confuses the mind.

Once an injury's cause has been understood, the exploration for recovery techniques can begin. The answers could be obvious or require a considerable amount of systematic searching. To be safe, with each new approach (manipulation, stretch, exercise, use of an outboard tool), do less, and do it more slowly and carefully, than you think you can, until you are sure that the technique is appropriate to your problem and that you are performing it correctly and safely within your injured limits. **Remember the 80% Rule:** In recovery, only do 80 percent of what you think you can safely do until, at least, one week after you feel fully recovered. There is nothing more frustrating than finally feeling great again, going for the gold prematurely and winding up back in the black and blue.

THE PAIN OF RECOVERY

Until you do feel fine again, a helpful limiter to your physical activity is pain. Yes, it distracts, but it is also a guide. The pain of injury lets you know when you're doing too much, doing too little, or sedentarily lounging in a harmful position, all of which can make the problem worse. Conversely, when using a helpful recovery technique, the pain of recovery defines the degree to which you can safely work and improve.

Though there is an obvious difference between these two—one feels harmful and one feels helpful—they are joined at the hip. The pain of recovery, which should be employed only in moderation, can, if you become impatient and push too hard through it, lead you, in an unwitting instant, across that razor's edge to the harsh pain of reinjury. This transition will leave you physically shocked and cognitively dismayed to realize what you've just done. If this happens, add a good few days to a couple of weeks to your getting back to normal.

HOW LONG IT TAKES

The most determining factor in how long an injury recovery will take is the degree and complexity of the injury in relation to the physical fitness of the injured. Generally, the more fit and healthy you are, the quicker you can recover.

Closely on these heels, however, are the recovery techniques themselves. Without the right tools, used in the right ways, you may never recover as far as possible, no matter how fit you may be.

Calm. Clarity. Diligence. Patience. Perseverance. These, when combined with Education and Safety, will always serve you well.

THE TOOLS IN THE WORKSHOP

The main thrust of exercise-related physical recovery lies in three things: flexibility, strength and massage. Various outboard paraphernalia—bandages, braces, tape—are sometimes indispensable to the safe introduction of the first two after an injury. Massage also has outboard equipment that can offer great relief under the right conditions.

MASSAGE GEAR

Along with fingers, hands and other body parts, there are numerous rollers, balls, and other tools of curious design, in various sizes, shapes and materials, available to use when massaging sore, knotted muscles. Though I will not rate them here (to some extent, it is a matter of taste), there are a couple of things to keep in mind when choosing such an accomplice.

First, size. Does it effectively cover the area of your concern? Is it specific enough to get into where you need it most? Does it feel beneficial?

As for shape, rollers that are broad and flat work well for many larger muscle groups, though some people prefer rollers with a more contoured surface. For smaller muscle groups, balls and other rounded objects are often more helpful. If what you're using leaves you wanting more, or less, look around and try something else.

The importance of the material used is absolute. Remember that muscle is meat and meat can be macerated and bruised, particularly when pressed between a hard object and hard bones. Any hard object employed—something made of wood or a baseball—that doesn't have any give to it should be used with great care. Especially when using considerable pressure (body weight is normally used), the consistency of the tool can make the difference between recovery and collateral injury.

Even with hands-only massage, using fists, knuckles, elbows to press the matter home might be something to avoid, for the same reason mentioned previously. Bones are actually harder than the materials used in the hardest outboard massage tools and are quite capable of bruising and macerating muscle, fascia, tendon and ligament. It might be easier to use bones, rather than fingers, from the power of giving point of view, but it can be detrimental to the recipient, complicating the injury already at hand.

When using any type of massage, think before you act. Even when you're sure of your actions, less can be more. Proceed with caution.

ICE AND HEAT

Ice and heat are both easy to use and very effective. Both reduce pain, both do a good job, and both have their moments to shine.

When you've got inflammation at the site, ice is your pal (minimum 30 minutes). Ice will reduce any unnecessary supersizing, or, at least, give some stiff resistance to its increase. Heat, however, is not generally recommended with inflammation. It may actually encourage excess inflammation or slow down its departure when it's time to go.

Dry heat, either electrically or chemically produced, shines where ice doesn't. Ice is generally not as comfortable to bear as heat and, as it melts, is prone to sweating and dripping on furniture and clothing, and must be (frequently) replenished. At home, at rest, electric heating pads (follow directions carefully) go as long as you want them to.

On the move, ice doesn't travel well attached to the body, but heat generating adhesive patches (plasters) can make the impossible possible. There have been times in my life, particularly one spring tour performing in Europe, and one night of heavy bartending in New York, when I could not even have risen from my bed without a Johnson and Johnson Back Plaster firmly attached and baking across my lower back.

In the first case, my lower spine was flirting with the idea of serious injury, but the show must go on. I'd never missed a performance in my life and wasn't about to start. For several days, I had to pay careful, diligent attention to stabilizing the situation, warming up cautiously and thoroughly before each performance. My meager supply of plasters ran out quickly, but they got me over the hump. I managed to avoid catastrophe and finish the tour. No one, onstage or off, ever caught on I was suffering.

In the second case, I was in much worse condition, recovering from the same catastrophe fully played out. Though I'd not been able to stand erect for several days, I needed the work that night and had taken the job. The plaster mitigated the pain enough to get to my feet and me out the door.

The event proved very popular, the drinks were free, and we were slammed hard—fast, loud, furious, people packed four deep, everybody calling out, wanting service right now, for six chaotic hours. I made it through and kept a pace at least equal to my fellow gin slingers, with no noticeable harm to my back, but, the moment my shift finished—Uungh! Was I sore!

Though I missed no more work and my recovery continued, I imagine I slowed it down a bit with my premature return to the labor force. Notwithstanding, I would be a less reliable, poorer, and, occasionally, feebler man were it not for these capsacin-based plasterers of backs.

When using any such heat patches, pay attention to the active ingredients. While most only topically ease the pain without actually helping the healing process, capsacin (also spelled capsicum, capsium) have been shown to increase blood flow to the area, which assists healing. Look into it yourself.

The more affluent among us may insist that heat is best when it does sweat and drip, as with steam rooms and Jacuzzis. Add dry saunas to the mix, and you have the never-ending controversy between wet and dry heat—which is better—that I've been hearing as long as I can remember. Having seldom had access to any of these on a regular basis, I must remain, in this case, uncharacteristically without an opinion.

I do, however, know a wet heat solution that is wonderful. It was taught to me by a dancer from Holland I spent time with, while she was studying in New York. All you need is a bathtub and hot running water.

Most people, she explained, fill the tub first and then get in. Five minutes later, they are no longer warm, for the water was not that hot to begin with, but only felt so by contrast to the temperature of the skin.

In her method, you get in the tub before you turn the water on, then continue turning up the heat as your body acclimates to the rising temperature of the water and the tub fills. Take it as hot as you safely can, as deep as you safely can, and stay in as long as you safely can.

It's an amazing thing. You soak, you sweat (keep a cold drink handy), and, if you last long enough, your pain will be relieved down to the marrow of your bones. You will have to dry off at least twice when you get out, as your body will sweat again after the initial drying.

Unless I have the good fortune of a Japanese bath, or a soak in the joy of a hot spring, if I am going to bathe, as opposed to shower, the method mentioned here is the one I prefer by far. It has been a faithful and constant defender against the slings and arrows of outrageous torture that so often assault the battered bastions of my muscles, sinews and bones.

BANDAGING, BRACES AND TAPE

These three essentials are used for the same purpose, which is to help support, stabilize and, where necessary, inhibit the range of motion of an injured area. As there are many different ways to be injured and many different configurations to our muscles and bones, one of these might be better used for one part of the body, one for another.

Bandaging (the supportive, fabric stretch type) can be used to wrap everything, from joints to long muscles and their attachments. The good thing about such bandaging is its ability to stretch, offering solid support—but not absolute constriction—to the injured area.

Done properly, bandaging will still allow the muscle to expand and contract comfortably throughout the body, preventing pinches, burns and strains where the unwrapped part of the muscle, which is completely free to expand, borders the wrapped area, which expands to the degree necessary for safe function, within the flexible support of the bandage.

The difficulty with bandaging is getting the tension even throughout, from beginning to end, and getting it to stay in place. Too tight in one spot, too loose in another, and the old injury can be renewed or a new, collateral injury can be born. When the muscle flexes and its natural expansion is restricted too much in one area, it tends to exert extra pressure into the unrestricted area, possibly causing harm.

To further complicate things, joints and muscles, when in use, change shape a lot. This means the pressure is constantly changing, at different rhythms, on every band of the wrapping, at every point along the band. Combine this fact with the pull of gravity and centrifugal force, and you've got the trifecta of slipping bandages. In my experience, regardless of how perfectly the bandaging has been applied, unless you're taking it easy, sooner or later, it is going to slip. Once slipped, it becomes, at least, less effective and, possibly, useless.

The one place where bandaging, in my opinion, perhaps does the best job is around the torso, in the case of cracked ribs, a strain to the muscles attached to the ribs, or an injury to the lower portion of the lats (*latissimus dorsi*, the large triangular muscles in the upper back that work primarily with the shoulders). Properly bandaged, movement of the area is usually quite restricted, minimizing slippage, and the quality of supportive flexibility in the bandaging is well attuned to the needs of the ribcage as it expands and contracts during breathing.

One could argue, however, that, even in this scenario, certain types of tape might do as good a job or better. Tape can be your best friend. It just depends on what kind of friend you need and what kind of tape you've got.

In my experience, a good sport tape is more versatile than either bandaging or braces. What I mean by sport tape, as there are at least two very different tapes currently being sold under that moniker, is the thinner, less sticky, slightly stretchy version of adhesive tape. Cut from the same cloth, where adhesive tape adheres determinedly and stretches nary a millimeter, sport tape stretches modestly and evenly, offering consistent support and a comfortable degree of flexibility.

Used to wrap an injured area in the same fashion as bandages, unless exposed to considerable moisture (an external water source or a continued heavy sweat), sport tape stays put and doesn't loosen. Nor does it put up a fight when you take it off, reducing the stress of pulling it from the injured area, reducing the burn on the skin and the loss of body hair at the sight (for the hirsute among us). Often, a little strip of sport tape can be used as effectively, at much less expense, as a pinpoint brace (see the following paragraph on braces). Also, sport tape can be used to assist bandages, bandaging and braces, as an extra emphasis in one spot, or by taping the seams of the bandaging together, or the edges of the brace to the skin, to inhibit slippage.

Relatively new to the scene, Kinesio tape (from kinesiology, the study of muscles and the mechanics of human motion) is similar to sport tape in its consistency and intent but is applied differently. Available in several degrees of thickness (differentiated by colors), rather than wrapping around an injury, it is applied along the lines of the presumably injured muscles, adhering them, to some extent, to the muscles on either side. Both this and the less stretchable consistency of the tape along the muscles are designed to give extra support and, I would think, a degree of extra warmth (as the body warms up) to the affected area.

I have not yet had occasion to use Kinesio tape, but, if you watched much of the 2012 Summer Olympics, you will most likely have seen its day-glo bright strips prominently displayed on the arms, shoulders, legs, fronts and backs of many of the competing athletes.

Braces, used primarily for joint injuries at the ankle, knee, wrist and elbow, are made in numerous shapes, sizes, and degrees of thickness. Many have holes at the outer bend of the joint or reinforcing pads and straps built into them. Some severely restrict movement, others merely give extra support.

Understandably, the thicker, reinforced, strapped braces are more restrictive than the lighter ones, which are about three times as thick as an Ace bandage (Ace makes braces as well). All that I have seen marketed to the general public come in various sizes, usually S, M, and L, but some are cutting production to two less distinct sizes, S/M and M/L. There are also braces that I have only seen dispensed by doctors. Of the heavier sort, some seem designed for a more specific intent than general joint rehabilitation.

Many thinner braces, and some thicker ones, are pre-formed and slip on over the foot or hand. Others wrap around to be secured by Velcro, especially such braces for the foot, ankle, calf and wrist and pinpoint braces.

I have never used anything more than the thinner, less restrictive (and less supportive) braces throughout my career, regardless of the degree of my injury (strains, dislocations, neural problems, tears). However, one must take into account one's general physical condition, training and ability to recover when assessing this statement. Were I in poorer shape, or less able to govern my recovery, the stronger, more restricting and supportive braces might have done me better.

There is a relatively new brace on the market, designed to support the muscles of the calf and help them remain securely attached to their bones. It is called a shin guard and was designed, I believe, to counter the evil of shin splints (see following section). If I were to use them, as every calf is different, I would go for the wrap around version with Velcro straps, to get a more uniform support, rather than the slip on pre-formed model. Seeing them successfully used, I imagine similar braces for the thigh, upper arm and forearm are also available or in the offing.

Another fairly recent innovation is the pinpoint brace, a half-inch wide or so wrap around a brace that attaches with Velcro, allowing as little or much pressure on the point of pain as one desires. It is a very useful tool for that nagging spot whose pain is relieved with just a bit of pressure. Usually the result of a small strain near an attachment of tendon to bone, or a knot in one small part of a muscle, this type of pinpoint pain is commonly found at the wrist and above and below the elbows and knees, though it can occur in the middle of a big muscle in the middle of a long bone (hamstring, calf, etc.).

The main thing about braces is that you feel more secure and comfortable moving with the injury. If wearing a brace is causing you more pain, it may be too tight, too restrictive, or not formed in a way that accommodates your body. (Though I have known numerous people who have happily worn a knee brace with a open hole at the kneecap, that design has proven consistently painful for me.) Find what suits your needs.

There is one silly thing I have heard, many times now, about wearing these braces, and it blows me away that thinking human beings so readily accept it as fact or that any educated person would give such simplistic advice in the first place. Numerous people have confided in me, over the years, when I have recommended wearing a brace to protect an injury, that they have it, on good authority, that wearing a brace for an injury leads to an addiction to wearing that brace. In other words, once accustomed to wearing the brace, one will never feel secure again without wearing it, regardless of complete recovery in the injured area.

What I would say to that cannot be printed here.

I will say that I have used braces, as needed, throughout my life and they have kept me going when, without them, I have no doubt I would have torn myself up (or torn myself up worse). I wear them as long as necessary and am always delighted to finally leave them off. It has been my experience that, when I don't feel the pain (a good sign of healing), I forget to put the brace on, no matter how long I've been using it. (I do try to remember to wear it a few more days, however, as the first pain-free day rarely means I'm completely healed.)

The only thing I can think of that might lead to an addiction to wearing a brace on a healthy joint would be a psychological compulsion in the individual and this, I believe, might be mitigated by strong, reassuring advice, on good authority, against psychological addiction. If such counseling proved ineffective, one might consider the problem lies deeper than a physical injury and a supportive brace.

HEADS UP

Though I can neither list nor imagine every different way the muscles, tendons, ligaments, joints, nerves and bones of the human body can be injured in physical activity, or from the lack thereof, various symptoms bear hallmarks that can guide you to the heart of most any problem. The injuries listed next offer a broad range of symptoms and solutions that, comprehensively, will give you a good foundation from which to explore those nefarious aches and jolting pains that become so peculiarly your own.

So, when you're hurt, examine the injury, figure out what's wrong and, unless surgery is required, in a timely manner work toward recovery—intelligently, with rest, support, ice and heat, massage, flexibility and strength rehab and lots of: **Caution! Follow the 80% Rule! Patience! Less Can Be More!**

Now, let's start looking at body parts.

THE NECK AND THE SHOULDERS

In physical training, I have rarely seen neck injuries that are restricted to the neck alone. By this, I mean injuries in which restricted movement, pain and relief of pain are only found from the neck up. Most involve the shoulders and the upper back as well. Still, there are one or two.

NECK INJURIES

Particularly susceptible to isolated injury and pain are the numerous smaller, overlapping, multi-layered muscles on the back and sides of the neck, found from just behind the ears to the spine of the neck (the cervical vertebra). Some of these muscles reach from the skull to the vertebrae and collarbones, others from the vertebrae to the ribs and collarbones. These muscles can freeze up from overuse, under-use, the stress of repeated motion, of lack of motion, habitual poor support and mental anxiety.

SYMPTOMS

1. A sharp, ripping burn up the side of the skull, when quickly turning the head to one side or the other

2. A dullish, nagging soreness or tightness, possibly throbbing, felt along one or both sides of the back of the neck

3. An electric shock, or sharp pain, when the head is placed in, or moves through, certain positions

4. Numbness

5. Any combination of these

ASSESSMENT

Felt primarily when muscles are tired, stiff, or dehydrated, the searing pain of symptom 1 suggests that at least one muscle involved in the rapid movement was either unwilling or unready to perform and did not stretch, or stretch enough, to facilitate the motion. As with a chain, this freeze-up causes the most stress and pain where the linkage is weakest, in this case from the connections at the base of the skull up through the broader, thinner muscle and fascia of the skull itself.

If you're lucky, the whole thing is just a fluke and will go away in a few minutes. If not, that area of your head could remain sore and susceptible to reinjury for days. What's more, it could be merely a side effect of deeper muscular problems (symptom 2) or unduly pressured nerves involving the vertebrae and discs of the neck (symptoms 3 and 4), either of which could be pre-existing or occur simultaneously with the event.

WHAT TO DO

Massage: For immediate relief, use acupressure (see **The Role of Acupressure**, from **Getting Involved**, chapter IX).

For symptom 1, start pressing up from the base of the skull into the scalp. Also, pressure applied along the base of the skull seems to have a strong effect on related structures in both the head and neck. A tennis ball can be very useful here (see **Gravity Driven Acupressure: Tennis Ball and Body Weight**, from **The Neck and Shoulders**).

Lie flat on your back, knees bent, feet on the floor. Place the tennis ball under your neck, just below the base of the skull, along the line of pain. This is a good place to start for two reasons: You want to work your way into the most painful area, not begin on it, and the natural curve of the neck, rising from the floor, allows one to easily control the degree of pressure from the ball placed in this position.

Without lifting the head, reach back and use your fingers to rotate the ball downward from the skull, toward the neck, while pushing it up under the base of the skull itself, until it supports the weight of the head (if you're bald or play pool, this downward spin puts a little "English" on the cue).

This oppositional rotation helps lengthen the neck—and therefore the injured area—as you bring the ball into the base of the skull. Lengthening the area in this passive manner encourages the tighter muscles to relax, helps relieve any undue pressure on the discs between the neck's vertebrae and makes one aware of a longer, more supportive alignment.

If you've got the ball well placed, you'll feel the pain of recovery emanating from that pressure point up through all of the affected area on the skull down into the worst of the injured muscles in the neck. Rotate the head, as necessary, to relegate both the point of application and the pressure. (Some people may find that using two tennis balls, the second on the other side, mirroring the first, offers more effective support and an easier control of the pressure.)

Do not use this position for more than a few minutes at a time, regardless of how helpful it feels. With the neck passively pulled out long, related structures may overreact to an injurious degree, completely unnoticed until you start to move and the painful truth is revealed. **Remember the 80% Rule.**

You can continue, however, for a considerable length of time, with the following modifications.

Roll the tennis ball down into the neck itself, allowing your normal degree of curvature to return. If the heightened curvature decreases the pressure from the ball too much to be effective, roll up a small towel, tightly, or take a small pillow and place it under the base of the skull. Then use your fingers, on the sides of your head, to rotate the passive back of your neck out longer (rotating the chin toward the chest). The towel holds the neck in this longer pull, while allowing it to relax as needed. Also, unless you're using a pillow, the back of the head stays in the same line as the back, flat on the floor. This is a less stressful position from which to work.

You may find relief with the head squared to the shoulders; you might feel even better with it turned to one side; perhaps what you need involves bringing the chin down toward one side of the chest or the other. Search carefully. Search thoroughly.

Movement: After the initial burning of symptom 1 is relieved, some gentle exploration of the movements of the head may be incorporated into the massage, depending on the degree of the injury. Try moving the chin slightly up and down, and in small circles at differing heights, before turning the head side to side. Once the uninjured ROM is defined, you will have a clearer picture of what stretches and strengthening can best effect a recovery.

Stretches: It's always best to begin with stretches in which the neck participates, but is not the central focus. Whenever possible, get a little blood flowing and warm the injured area up a bit before getting into its specifics.

If I were going for a full workout (and planning to help my neck along the way), I would begin with most or all of the active stretches in chapter VIII, before proceeding to the following **Head and Shoulder Rolls** section.

If I were relaxed and pursuing relief, I would begin with the **Standing Hangover Stretch**.

STANDING HANGOVER STRETCH

1. Stand with the feet at hip-width or slightly wider, toes forward, knees slightly bent (Photo 188).

2. Supporting with your belly, roll your head forward and down, and let the body follow, rounding down vertebra by vertebra (Photo 189). Keep your weight in your heels.

3. Once at the bottom, relax and breathe, deeply and slowly, inhaling from the lower back all the way up into the shoulders, exhaling from the shoulders down through the lower back. Be sure to relax your neck.

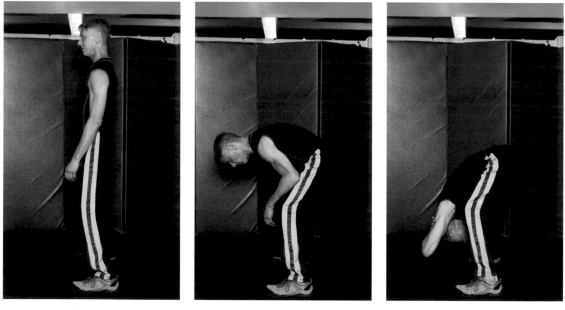

PHOTO 188   PHOTO 189   PHOTO 190

Don't think about stretching, just relax (the belly still supports!) and focus on your breathing. Remain there for a few seconds up to a minute or so.

If your neck isn't too sore, bend your arms behind your head. Place your left hand on your right shoulder and your right hand on your left and continue to hang (Photo 190).

4. When ready to rise, take a deep breath, then exhale slowly, using your belly, as you roll the body up, one vertebra at a time, the head being the last to lift. (Remember, it's always safer to keep the knees slightly bent as you roll up.)

Hanging over thusly, with the knees slightly bent and belly supporting, allows the entire back of the body to open up, from the calves through the hamstrings to the lower back and, from there, on up through the spine, the long muscles of the back and into the shoulders, neck and head.

The **Half Lotus Variation** (chapter VIII) makes a great next stretch. The forward stretch, begun from the lower back and hips, reaches out through the entire spine to full extension, and offers benefits to the muscles of the upper back and shoulders as well (remember, they're all related), as you work into the neck. The work to the sides, focusing on the middle and upper back and shoulders, warms up and stretches everything connected to the neck, secondarily providing warmth, mild stretch and stability challenges to the neck itself.

Follow this up with **Flutter-Bys** (chapter VIII), which finishes with a seated, straight-legged, nose to knees (or farther) pullover stretch. When performed with flexed feet, this works everything from the bottom of the toes through the back of the skull. The head stretching forward and down assists the discs between the vertebrae in their alignment. Since the head follows, not leads, one can easily govern the extent to which the neck participates, keeping well within the 80% limit.

Head and Shoulder Rolls are most beneficial when the body has been warmed up. It is important, while isolating the working muscles of the shoulders and neck, to keep the rest of the body properly aligned, supported and unmoving.

HEAD AND SHOULDER ROLLS

1. Sit or stand up straight, belly supporting, shoulders in place, back of the neck long.

2. Keep the rest of the body perfectly still (don't forget to breathe). Rotate one shoulder forward (Photo 191). If the neck is sore on one side, starting with the opposite shoulder will most likely work best.

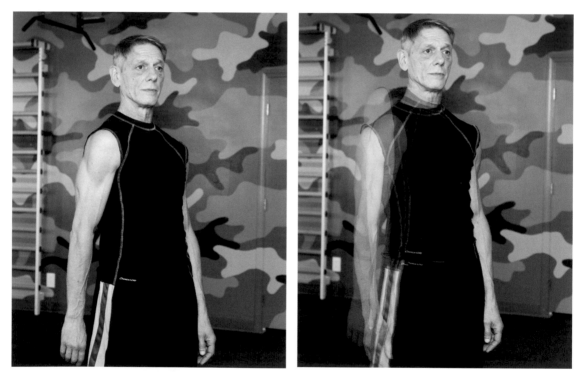

PHOTO 191

Keeping the elbow forward of the torso, continue rotating your shoulder, in a full circle, up (Photo 192) back (Photo 193), down and forward (Photo 194), through your full ROM, past the torso and again to the front.

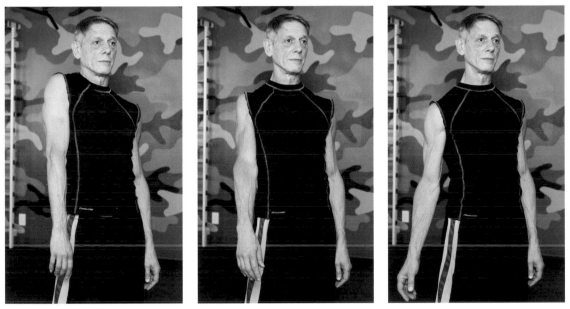

PHOTO 192   PHOTO 193   PHOTO 194

Eight repetitions one shoulder, then do the other. Use your muscles, don't just move in thoughtless motion. Squeeze them. Please them. If you work full range, you'll find that, when the shoulder passes the body at the bottom of the circle, it actually presses lower into the body than when it is in normal alignment. It may be hard at first, isolating a moving shoulder from an unmoving body, but keep it up and success will come.

If there is a burn or pinch in the neck or shoulder in one spot of the rotation, reduce the ROM and the speed in that shoulder until the sensation softens. It mainly occurs as the "up and back" rotation transitions to the "back and down," just behind the midline of the body.

If there is a painful click through this position, or any position, the symptom may be different but the safety measures are the same. (In most cases, you'll find that reversing the motion reduces or eliminates the sensation.)

3. Beginning with the first shoulder, rotate each, for eight repetitions, in the opposite direction (back, up, forward and down). Again, try to keep the elbow forward of the torso. (This reverse direction of movement is a little tougher to perform properly.)

4. Now, rotate one shoulder forward, up (Photo 195) and back, and hold it to the back (Photo 196) while rotating the other forward, up and back to join it (an extreme version of the army's "Chest out! Shoulders back!") (Photo 197).

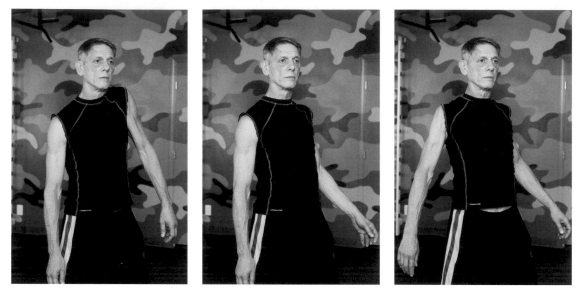

PHOTO 195   PHOTO 196   PHOTO 197

The first shoulder then reverses, rolling up, forward and down, then remains forward and down as the second shoulder follows. Four repetitions leading with the right, four left.

5. Now, rotate the shoulders simultaneously forward (Photo 198), up (Photo 199), and back (Photo 200), then up, forward and down, for four repetitions.

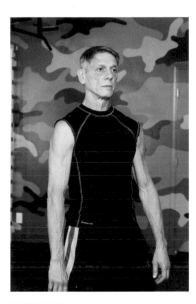

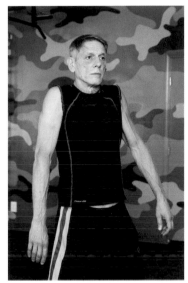

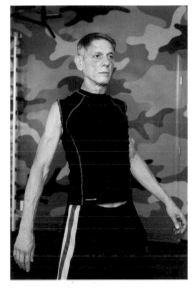

PHOTO 198   PHOTO 199   PHOTO 200

6. Return the shoulders to neutral position (proper alignment) and remain strong and still. With the back of the neck long, bring the chin toward the chest at an even and moderate pace (Photo 201).

As soon as it reaches its limit, lift it right back up toward the sky (Photo 202), then down again and up, and so on, for eight repetitions.

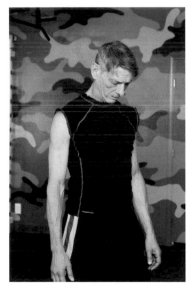

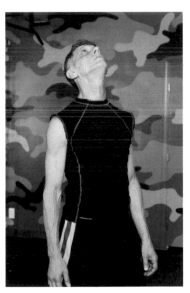

PHOTO 201   PHOTO 202

When you take the head back, remember to keep the neck engaged and lifting, as opposed to just dropping the head behind the back loosely and crunching all them pretty little discs. Conversely, be sure you're not just jutting your chin out, forward and up, but are actually laying into the muscles of the back of the neck.

7. Bring your head back to normal alignment. Now, turn your face to the right and left. Keep the back of the neck long, chin level (Photo 203).
Smooth and even pace. Eight repetitions.

8. Again bring the chin to the chest (Photo 204)
From here, roll the head around to one side, as if bringing the ear to the shoulder (Photo 205).

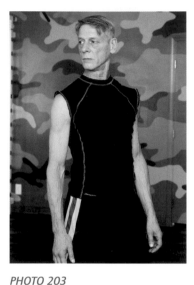 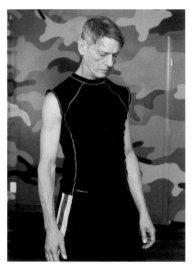 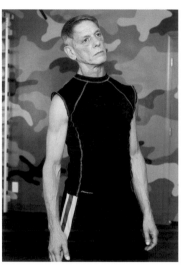

PHOTO 203   PHOTO 204   PHOTO 205

Refrain from turning the head (the face). Try to keep your face forward and both shoulders firmly grounded.

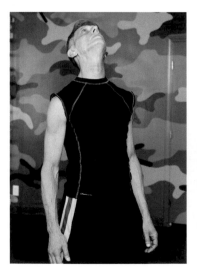 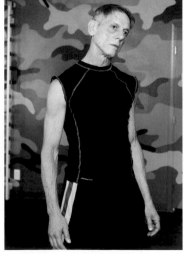

Continue rolling the head around the side, to the back (Photo 206) (face to the sky), around the other side (Photo 207) and forward again, to the chin to the chest. Smooth, even circles, four of them each side, nice and calm and controlled. Getting into the pain a little is okay, but remember the 80% Rule.

PHOTO 206   PHOTO 207

If, in going to one side, you feel a burn, a cramp or sharp pain, especially as you pass a particular point, decrease the ROM as you pass through that spot and slow down the speed.

If you still feel the pain, and you cannot mitigate it sufficiently by clipping your ROM, leave that direction alone for a few days. Just do the neck rolls that begin to the other side. The affected area responds more reasonably, in most cases, when rolled through from the opposite direction.

This problem usually occurs when the head is just behind the shoulder, and the muscles in the back of the neck, on that side, are most contracted, and their related discs are under the most pressure.

HAND-ASSISTED NECK STRETCH

THE STANDARD APPROACH (NOT SHOWN)

1. Reach across the top of your head and place your hand on the other side of your skull.

2. Pull the head in that direction, ear to the shoulder, thus stretching the opposite **side** of the neck.

This stretch is regularly performed by thousands of well-intentioned people every day. In virtually every case, the head is pulled directly to the side. From my experience, with the exception of a very specific problem or two (too many overhead presses? too many harassing stresses?), this position is only moderately beneficial, and, for some, potentially harmful.

The thing is, most of the muscles available to stretch lie not directly on the sides of the neck, but in its rear quadrants, between the sides and the back. Therefore, pulling the head directly to the side, rather than focusing directly on the bulk of the muscles available to stretch, turns a good bit of that potential stretch into some serious lateral pressure on the vertebrae and discs. This can not only compress the discs to a harmful degree, it can also cause the vertebrae and discs to misalign, neither of which a normal person would want to happen.

Considering this, it seems to me that bringing the head somewhat forward, as it is pulled to the side, would make more sense. The muscles get all their stretch; the vertebrae and discs are more protected.

VARIATION IN D MAJOR

1. Reach over the top of the head and place the hand on the opposite rear quadrant of the crown of the skull (Photo 208).

2. Using gravity more than strength, ease the head slightly forward and over to the side, until a good stretch is achieved.

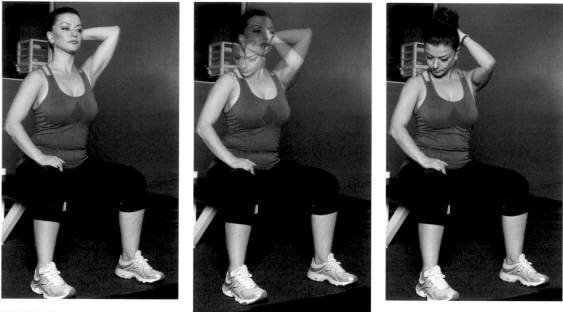

PHOTO 208   PHOTO 209

I would suggest that you don't actually have to pull at all, in most cases, to get all the stretch you should. Just the weight of the hand across the head is usually enough. Too much might, *might* feel nice at first, but it also might bite you in the end.

3. Very slowly, try turning the face to the same side, by comfortable degrees, and see how this affects the focus of the stretch (Photo 209). The head may also be rotated more forward to the same purpose, but be very slow and cautious in doing so.

4. Don't stay there too long. Thirty seconds max. As with certain other positions, staying there too long could cause other problems, which may lie unnoticed until you release. Once you've crossed that razor's edge, for even half a second, you will most likely have opened a new can of worms that could take weeks to consume.

Any of these techniques may be employed, whether warmed up or not, whenever you have the time and feel the need. A sore neck can be very distracting, and the relief found in a few seconds of massage, or stretch, here and there, may be enough to get you through a tough day.

Exercises: The best exercise for a sore neck is continuous strong support and proper alignment, though **Lat Pull-Downs** and **Headbangers** (chapter VI) may give some relief as well. Along with this, truly and thoughtfully engaging all the pertinent muscles while performing the **Head and Shoulder Rolls**, a couple of times a day, is your best shot.

If you're not too sore, incorporating neck therapy into your normal workout is a great way to go. Take things a little slower, if you need to, and always be aware of your neck and shoulder alignment.

NECK AND SHOULDER INJURIES

PART ONE

Though the pain of this next one is felt purely from the base of the neck to the skull, its cause and solution are found with the shoulders. It is a good example of how one small muscle's injury can affect one's bigger physical world. It also reminds me that, regardless of how experienced one may be, there's always something new to learn.

Presumably rare, I have only seen this injury twice in my life, both in the last year. One was mine and the other belonged to a hardworking water polo player. Both born of repetitive stress (though I've no doubt it could be caused by too much immediate stress), the primary muscle affected is one whose only real job is to lift the shoulder blades. That doesn't sound like much until you realize the shoulder blades are involved in virtually every movement the arms make. It's a shorter muscle, running from the top four vertebrae of the neck to the top inside edge of the shoulder blade. It doesn't connect directly to the base of the skull. (If you're curious, it's called the *levator scapulae*.)

In my case, I supported a heavy book in my left hand, for hours at a time (elbow at my side, bent to 90 degrees, book open before me at my waist, face rotated down to see it), over three days of intense study. This put a lot of unnoticed stress in the left rear quadrant of my neck. Though I would get a little sore while reading each day, I'd do a few stretches, a little exercise and not think much about it.

On the fourth day, I awoke with a steady, annoying ache in the area. Though the pain was livable, it would not be ignored, and I soon discovered that it could flare, exponentially, with one wrong move.

SYMPTOMS

I soon couldn't raise my shoulder without intense pain, nor could I carry any considerable weight in my left hand, without that part of my neck feeling sore and strained. Any number of smaller, lighter movements caused the muscle to engage secondarily and complain loudly about the motion.

Something as simple as reaching for a glass, or lifting a fork, could sharply remind me of what I'd done to myself. Over the next few days, I was really surprised to see just how invasive this injury had become. It was clear that, though I'd had a wide variety of injuries over the years, I'd found a new one, and it was mine all mine. Oh, joy!

In the case of the water poloist, the injury came by a different road, that of working vigorously, for long periods of time, day after day, with the arms above the shoulders. Sad to say, where I only hurt one side of my neck, she got them both.

It took some time, from when I first understood the nature of this injury, to figure out how to deal with it, though I found nothing to bring about a speedy recovery. It just came down to patience and proper care, doing my best to diminish the soreness, steadily though slowly, little by little every day.

ASSESSMENT

Overstressed muscles in the neck due to overworked shoulder blade.

WHAT TO DO

Stretches: Hold, for several seconds at a time, a strong downward (into the body)—and slightly back—rotation of the shoulder blades, simultaneously lifting strongly through the back of the neck.

Also helpful are the **Variation in D Major**, the (supine) **Shoulder Rotation and ROM** (chapter II), and the **Head and Shoulder Rolls**.

Massage: The same techniques prescribed for **neck injuries**, applied in slightly different locations. (The base of the skull does not figure as importantly for recovery in this injury, nor did I enjoy as much relief from acupressure, but that could be related to the severity and relative isolation of the injury itself.)

Movement: Conscientious alignment and support of the neck at all times, thoughtful placement and use of the shoulders and arms, whether active or at rest.

Exercises: From chapter VI, when possible (with reduced weight as necessary), try **Seated Upright Rows** and **Biceps Curls**—using a resistance band secured by the feet and locking the shoulders down,

Flies, both **Reverse** and **Chest**, with considerably reduced weight on the **Chest Flies** and maybe on the **Reverse**.

As your ROM begins to recover, **Lat Pull-Downs** and **Headbangers** become beneficial.

After a couple of days, I found I could do virtually all my regular workout, though there were places I had to consider (lower weight on my Bench Presses and Flies). On the upside, while my neck was warm, it felt pretty free. Of course, later on it would become tighter and more sensitive again, and I had to be careful how I slept.

I spent about six weeks recovering from that one. The water poloist, who had tried, as I had when I was younger, to keep playing and power through her injury, had a longer road.

PART TWO
Most neck and shoulder injuries are more comprehensive than those described already. The areas affected, both by pain and remedy, tend to be broader and more complex. There are so many moveable parts to the neck and shoulder assembly, so many smaller muscles reliant on the relative flexibility, strength and support of others around them, that virtually any injury to one part of the structure brings other parts into play. Though the specific qualities and locations of these injuries may vary, they are determined and dealt with in similar fashion.

SYMPTOMS
1. Tightness, soreness or a sudden shock along one or both sides of the back of the neck when you move, possibly in the vertebrae of the neck as well

2. Any of these three symptoms along the long ridge of muscle that reaches from the neck toward the shoulders (the *trapezius* muscle)

3. A line, or intermittent areas, of pain along the inside of one or both shoulder blades

ASSESSMENT
Though these things can be brought on by sudden occurrence or repetitive physical stress, the most common cause of these problems may be continued mental stress. Psycho-emotional tension. The harried harassments of daily life as we sometimes find it. The mind becomes agitated and the neck and shoulders tighten and lift (contract).

If they remain this way for any length of time, one enters the realm of Repetitive Stress Syndrome, where any particular motion, or postural proclivity, is repeated so often it causes injury. This reaction from daily stress, or something as innocuous as always sleeping on the same side of the body, can engender weeks of incredulous misery. The way things are carried—always with the same hand, always on the same shoulder—too much of any particular exercise, whether slow, fast, smooth, ballistic—all can work their repetitively stressed evils on the neck and shoulders.

Support and flexibility also have a huge impact. Allowing the shoulders to regularly slump forward, as part of your normal posture, overstretches—and, therefore, overstresses—the back of the shoulders, as well as adds compression to the discs of the neck, if the chin juts forward in compensation as it often does. Common in older people is a diminished ROM (particularly, reaching overhead), largely due to lack of regularly using their ROM. Especially as one ages, such a sedentary approach encourages joints to stiffen, and muscles and fat to coalesce into one big, tight mass, that puts the squeeze on all those otherwise happy joints and nerves.

WHAT TO DO

Deep breathing: Mental and emotional stress can eat you alive. Once they've got their hooks in you, they're hard to shed. Deep, relaxing breathing, however, can set you free.

You don't have to meditate, you don't have to sit in any curious posture, but you don't want to be curled up on the couch either. You'll do best with length and alignment. The idea is to have a free and open vessel into which the air may be drawn and expelled without obstruction.

Of course, sitting tall on the floor, with legs crossed in **Lotus** position, is fine if that's what you like. Sitting tall in a chair is fine, just support through your entire torso. If you're reclining onto a supporting surface (a couch?), a little external support for the lower back (a pillow, perhaps) will be useful to keep the lower back better supported.

When you're ready, inhale, slowly and steadily, from below the navel. The lower belly, expanding mildly, pulls the air into the bottom of the lungs. Continue to inhale and focus your mind exclusively on the air flowing in, as a jar fills with water, until you have a sense of near fullness. Then, begin a slow, measured exhale, keeping your relaxed, supported and aligned body lifted throughout.

Stay focused on your breathing. Breathe as slowly as you can. You may have to take a couple of quick breaths along the way until you develop a deeper breathing capacity.

When other thoughts float into your mind, don't let them distract you. Just concentrate on your breathing, and they will float right on out again. It may take a little practice to get this going, but it is aided, from the very beginning, by the physical act of deep breathing alone. As the mind will learn to calm the body, the body first, through deep breathing, will calm the mind.

You may sit and breathe in this manner for as long as you like, but as little as five minutes a day will, over a few weeks, make a huge difference in your ability to deal with mental and emotional stress. Practiced regularly, every day, the possibilities are endless. Really!

Movement: Clearly, with neck and shoulder problems, some movements or postures can be painful and, once identified, should be avoided. As always, focusing on proper structure and support will help greatly to clear things up, just as ignoring these will work to your debilitation. Habitual practices of standing, carrying, sleeping should be reviewed for contributing cause.

Massage: For the neck, see **Neck Injuries**. For pain extending from the neck along the ridge of the shoulder, define the line of pain by gently pressing or drumming the fingers along its length (use the opposite hand, reaching across the front of the body). Apply acupressure where and to the extent that it feels right. (If you choose to rub the muscle instead, back off of the pressure a little, for safety's sake.) If the pain is not along the top of the shoulder, but further into the back, use a foam roller or a tennis ball and let gravity do the work.

Regardless of where the pain is felt, it pays to explore the surrounding area for contributing causes. This means examining the neck, upper back and shoulder blades. The neck can be examined either with fingers or outboard pressure. For the upper back and shoulder blades, the best way I know is a tennis ball and body weight.

GRAVITY-DRIVEN ACUPRESSURE: TENNIS BALL AND BODY WEIGHT

1. Lie on the floor, on your back.

2. Bend one knee and, stabilizing with the foot, lean slightly to one side. Place a tennis ball under the pointed base of the lifted side's shoulder blade (Photo 210).

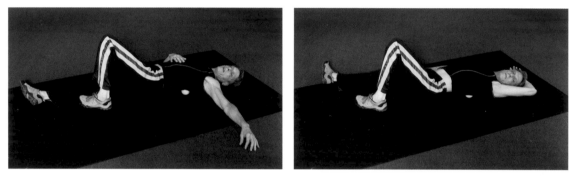

PHOTO 210   *PHOTO 211*

Lower the body onto the ball until the pressure is as you like it.

3. Without lifting your body, slide—slowly!—along the floor, causing the tennis ball to roll up along the inside edge of the shoulder blade. If there are contributing causes to your neck and shoulder problems, some, or all, are almost certain to lie along this path and the tennis ball will find them. When it does, you'll know it.

4. Upon reaching a contributing cause, remain there, with the ball applying pressure, for any part of two or three minutes, as along as it feels beneficial, before continuing your journey. A variation on this, which is sometimes helpful, is to **very slowly** rotate the affected arm around, through different positions, while the ball remains stationary (Photo 211). Ease the pressure a bit as you do so.

When you get to the top of the shoulder blade, roll the ball, as needed, out along the back of the shoulder, or in and up, into the neck.

Stretches: A safe way to begin is the **Shoulder Rotation and ROM** (chapter II). If performing this, slowly and gently, on the floor feels fine, you may increase the challenge by trying it on a bench or Swiss ball. Both of these offer a wider ROM, as the floor no longer inhibits movement to the back. Because of the Swiss ball's curve, which lifts through the center of the chest, it offers the greatest (yet also more stressful) opportunity to fully explore the shoulders' ROM.

SWISS BALL AND SHOULDER ROTATION

1. Lie on a large Swiss ball, on your back, feet wider than the hips, knees bent at 90 degrees, in line with the hips and toes. Keep the hips engaged and lifted. Belly presumably flat.

2. With the head supported comfortably on the ball (it is allowed to tilt back) align the peak of the ball's arch under the center of the chest, or as close as possible (this will be determined by the comfort of the neck). Adjust the legs and feet as necessary.

3. The arms flow in a full circle, full ROM (Photos 212, 213, 214),

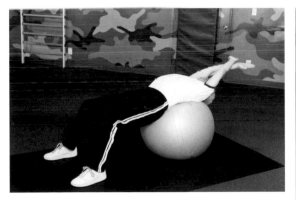

PHOTO 212

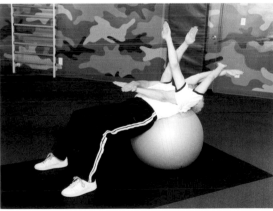

PHOTO 213

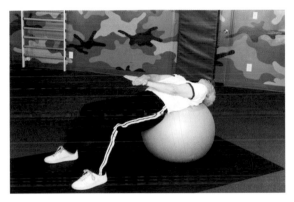

PHOTO 214

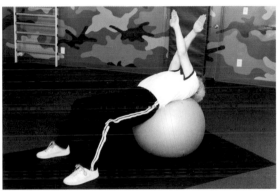

following the movements described in **Shoulder Rotation** and ROM (Photos 215, 216, 217).

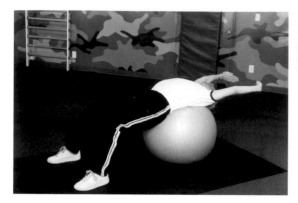

PHOTO 215

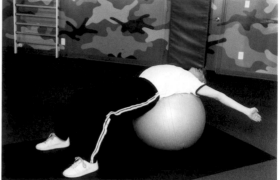

PHOTO 216

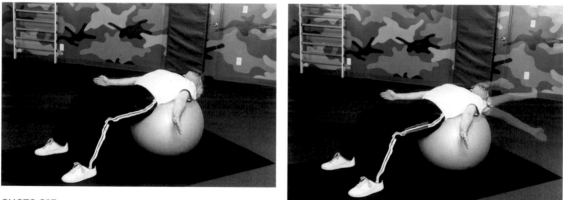

PHOTO 217

From here, the **Windmills**, **Side to Side**, and **Arm Circles** could be helpful, as well as the **Half Lotus Variation** (all in chapter VIII). Once you're warm, **Head and Shoulder Rolls** can be done.

Throughout your therapy, any whole-body stretches in which the neck and shoulders participate can be used. These are helpful particularly when the injured area is too sore to do much work on it directly, but not so sore that it cannot benefit from working together with the body in its entirety.

On a more passive note, the **Variation in D Major** can be used as often as you like. On a thoroughly passive note, there are a couple of relaxing postures that can really ease the situation.

Simply leaning back comfortably, or reclining entirely, and coupling your hands behind your head, can bring enormous comfort to the shoulders, upper back and neck. If you have the flexibility, reach farther across, behind your head, and try placing the left hand on the back of the right shoulder, and the right on the back of the left. Relax into that and see how you feel.

Also, whenever you're sitting, a tennis ball can be placed between the back of the chair and your shoulder (the pressure of the body against the chair holds it in place). While driving a car or commuting on public transportation, a well-placed tennis ball can make your journey a very pleasant one.

Exercises (all suggested are found in chapter VI): Lat Pull-Downs (watch your form!), **Seated Upright Rows, Headbangers** and **Reverse Flies**. The idea is to reset the proper alignment of the region, and rebuild a balanced support system, by getting the whole neighborhood working together again.

Biceps Curls, done standing with a resistance band, will be helpful. **Flies**, both flat and inclined, are useful (keep that neck long in the back)—with lighter weight as necessary—depending on the degree of pain and the 80% Rule.

Actually, with the exception of **Overhead Presses** and **Shrugs** (not shown) or other weightlifting contractions of the neck and shoulder junction (the *trapezius* muscle and friends), just about any upper-body or whole-body exercise should be fine, once you determine, cautiously, that it feels fine to perform it.

SHOULDER INJURIES

Closely related to **Neck and Shoulder Injuries**, though not the same, are **Shoulder Injuries**. Both have connection with the shoulder blades, but, where, in the first case, pain appears particularly in the neck and its junction with the inner shoulder, in the second it usually appears, also, at or near the outer end of the shoulder and its junction with the upper arm, and down into the shoulder blade.

Though the only, or primary, pain may be felt in one place, that doesn't necessarily mean that's where the (only) problem lies. With two very moveable joints in the area—the shoulder blade and the shoulder socket—and one joint moveable enough, where the tops of the shoulder blades meet the ends of the collarbones—and with so many muscles sharing responsibility for such a wide variety of movements, it seems whenever something's up with one of these guys, the whole neighborhood wants to get involved. Since this is the case, a brief introduction to the community might be in order.

Perhaps you've heard of the rotator cuff, as in, "The doctor says I tore my rotator cuff." The rotator cuff is a group of four muscles that are responsible for the stability of the shoulder joint. They stretch from the inner edge of the shoulder blade to wrap around the bone of the upper arm (the *humerus*) at the shoulder joint, the shallow ball and socket where the shoulder and upper arm join (three of them wrap from the back, one from the front). In other words, they're the muscles that hold it all together up there.

Surprisingly, these guys must also supply the thrust both for ballistic throwing and punching and for putting on the brakes at the end of such moves. Now, it seems to me, that this side of their lives— "Speed up! Slow down! Recoil and fire! Recoil and fire!"—would radically increase the simultaneous burden of stability and togetherness for which the rotator cuff is so primarily responsible. No wonder it gets so frequently torn.

Sharing this garment district with the rotator "cuff" is another piece of internal clothing, the shoulder girdle ("Does this dress make me look fat?"). Reaching from the spine of the neck and the upper back and from the upper ribs in front to hook up with the shoulder blades, this group of six muscles drive pretty much all the lifting, the squeezing back, the rounding forward and the bulk of the locking down of the shoulders.

Riding this turmoil out, like cowpokes on a bull, sit the three deltoid (delta-shaped) muscles, the kings of the mountain. On top of the shoulders and wrapping over the socket, into the upper arms, they do a lot of the lifting, pulling down and rotating of the arms.

Their friends, the biceps, the triceps, the *pectoralis major* and *minor* ("pecs," i.e., the chest) and others, also make personal investments in both the movements and stability of the shoulder joints. (Their share of the pie may not be as big, but it wouldn't be shoulder pie without them.)

So you see, the shoulders are a crowded place to live. It takes a lot of getting along to keep everyone happy, healthy and bursting with love. On the other hand, it takes very little to stir things up.

Let's see what happens when trouble breaks out.

SYMPTOMS

1. Sharp pain when the arm is lifted out and to the side of the body, at near or above the height of the shoulder (impingement syndrome)

2. Dull, sharp or nagging pain along the front, top or back of the shoulder

3. Pain along the upper arm, within or just below the deltoids; or underneath, just below or involving the armpit

4. Soreness or nagging pain along the side of the torso, underneath the shoulder joint

5. Soreness along the ridge of the shoulders or the inside or outside edges of the shoulder blades

ASSESSMENT

1. Impingement syndrome: The ends of the collarbones, as I mentioned, form a joint with the tops of the shoulder blades, immediately above the shoulder socket. Connected by ligaments, these bones perform a slight gliding movement as the arm and shoulder move through various positions. When they don't get it right, the ligaments, tendons or muscles feel the strain and the symptom becomes apparent.

   It can come from anywhere—the way you slept last night, repetitive stress, postural habits or one wrong move. Though the problem may feel extremely localized, it won't be. Something related got out of line, something somewhere was too relaxed or too tight.

   There will be some culpable muscles. They may be hiding out, but they will need to be found and brought to justice.

2-5. These can come from any of the same reasons as symptom **1**, but symptoms **2** and **3**, especially, can signal possible rotator cuff problems. There is one exercise designed specifically to combat this malady, shown in the following exercises.

WHAT TO DO

Massage: Use the same techniques as for the **Neck** and **Neck and Shoulders**. However, if there is pain along the side of the body, so that you have to lie on your side to use **Gravity Driven Acupressure**, a foam roller may prove easier to use than a tennis ball, as it provides additional support for the torso in this position, making it easier to relax the areas being massaged.

Movement: See **Neck and Shoulder Injuries**, **Part Two**.

Stretches: All those, in the order given, for **Neck and Shoulder Injuries**, **Part Two**, with the following considerations:

"In the order given" is especially important for impingement syndrome where, when lying down, one often has a greater ROM safely available, to help the recovery, than when standing.

Windmills, **Side to Side** and **Arm Circles** (chapter VIII) will almost definitely have to be slowed down—considerably—to safely work through the ROM. The ROM of the injured side may have to be abridged (80% Rule). If one shoulder feels fine, but the other must move slowly, move slowly with both. Don't lop-side your workout. If one direction doesn't feel right, don't work it with the injured shoulder, but you may with your good one, at a relaxed pace, to get the stretch.

The **Half Lotus Variation** (chapter VIII) can be very useful for the shoulders. Not only the beginning forward stretch that works around to the sides, but also when sitting and leaning to one side, as the other arm is raised out to the other side, then swung overhead.

Though the torso is vertical, leaning to the side changes the gravitational stress on the working shoulder and, even with impingement syndrome, movement that is painful when the torso is straight up may be pain free in this position. If the pain is merely lessened, and not enough to feel recuperative, lighten the load by folding the forearm in and bringing the hand close to the body, then think of pushing the elbow up and in, over the crown of the head, rather than reaching out long to the side with the arm extended.

There are two passive stretches, commonly seen, for the front and back of the shoulders, respectively.

WALL-ASSISTED PASSIVE SHOULDER STRETCH

1. Stand tall, face a wall up close, and reach out to the side with a straight working arm. Place the thumb side of the wrist against the wall.

2. Slowly rotate your chest away from the arm (gently, now) (Photo 218).

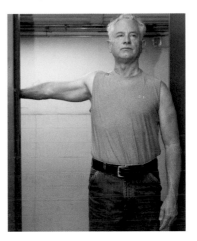

PHOTO 218

SELF-ASSISTED PASSIVE SHOULDER STRETCH

1. Lift the working arm up to shoulder height.

2. Take the back of the working arm, just above the elbow, with the opposite hand, and pull it across the front of your body at shoulder height (the relaxed elbow is approximately under the chin at this point) (Photo 219).

3. Press the (passive) working arm farther across and into the body, stretching the back of the shoulder (Photo 220) (take care not to let the working shoulder rise unintentionally). The passive forearm may remain extended or rest on the shoulder (each affects the stretch).

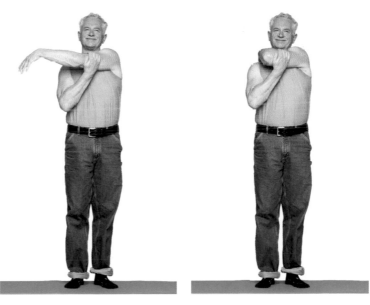

PHOTO 219   *PHOTO 220*

Though I use both of these stretches from time to time, it seems that they are easily overdone, which is to say that I have injured other muscles, in the immediate area, more than once, by going for a really good stretch in this manner. It may be because my shoulder muscles are already pretty flexible, and trained to various individual, fine-tuned movements, and either of these may offer a greater potential for destabilization in certain stressful positions. Or, it may just be that my zeal has outweighed my capability in these positions.

Whatever the reason for my trouble, from my experience, I would recommend to anyone a little extra care when using these two passive postures.

Relaxing with the hands behind the head seems to help anything in the region. Also, there is one more relaxing position I know that can really hit the spot.

COUCH-ASSISTED SHOULDER STRETCH

1. Sit back into a bench or a relatively firm couch, until your back is supported all the way, from the hips up. Lift tall through the crown of your head and support with your belly.

2. From the upper chest, arch slightly forward and up (a small, dense pillow in the middle of the back can help), and reach the arms out long to either side, along the top of the back of the couch, palms down. (If the back of the couch rises much higher than the middle of your shoulder blades, you may have to sit on a cushion, or two, to adjust the height.)

3. With arms fully extended, press your shoulders down into your body (Photo 221).

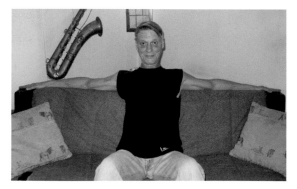

PHOTO 221

This produces a very relieving sensation that can reach from the inner shoulders all the way out through the fingertips. I've spent as long as 10 or 15 minutes at one time in this position and found nothing but positive results. Very relaxing after a long day.

For a sympathetic variation, rotate your arms and place the back of both hands against the back of the couch (Photo 222). Keep reaching out long, and keep the shoulder pressing down.

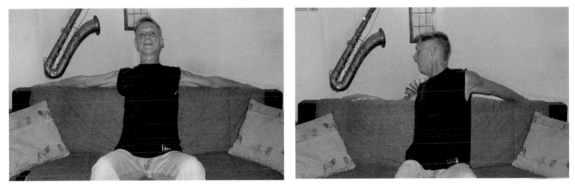

PHOTO 222   *PHOTO 223*

Now, leave one hand there, and use the other arm to rotate the body to the opposite side (Photo 223).

Exercises: All of the same found in **Neck and Shoulder Injuries**, **Part Two**, with a few additions. After **Lat Pull-Downs** and **Seated Upright Rows**, you might want to try the following.

DOWN-AND-OUT PRESS

1. Place a bench or a Swiss ball under a sturdy overhead bar or beam, such as a cable machine or a chin-up bar. Toss a resistance band over the top (the bar should pass from back to front, not side to side), grab the handles falling from either side, and have a seat. As you sit, the hands will be drawn overhead to a height determined by the length of the hanging band.

(With impingement syndrome, take the hands forward and up as you sit, rather than to the sides. If this is still painful, try folding the hands in near the chest, as you continue holding the handles, and let the arms be drawn up vertically above the body.)

2. Sit tall and support through your torso. Knees are wider than the hips, aligned with the feet and bent to no more than 90 degrees.

3. Press the shoulders firmly into the body and draw the backs of the wrists together over the crown of the head (Photo 224).

The elbows bend a bit to allow this. Keep them at this angle throughout the exercise.

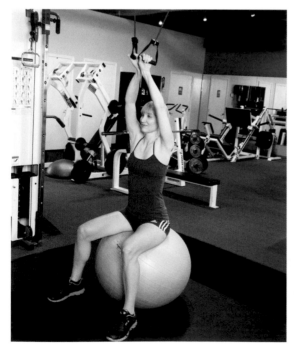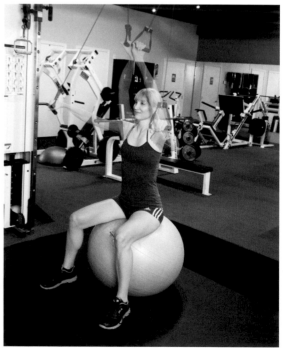

PHOTO 224

With a firm grip, press the wrists out and down, the arms—from the shoulders—out wide and down along with them (Photo 225), all the way down to your hips, palms facing in (as much as the band allows) (Photo 226).

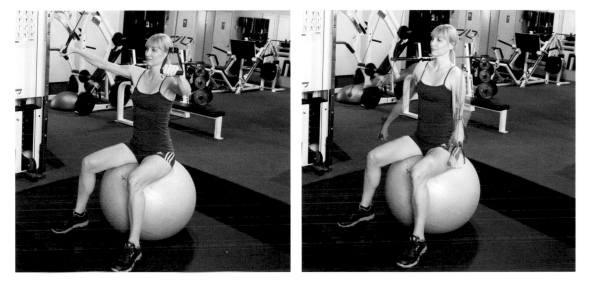

PHOTO 225

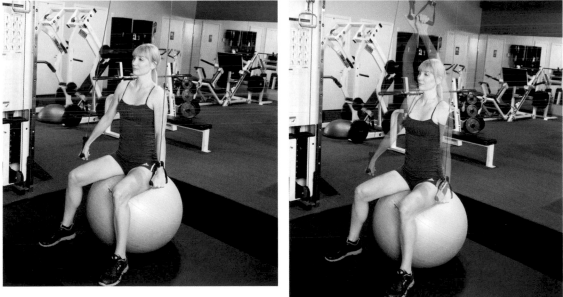

PHOTO 226

4. Keep the shoulders in place and allow the arms to be drawn back overhead by the contraction of the band, along the same path as possible.

Repetitions will vary, depending on the resistance of the band. Still, you should feel well worked by 20.

You will notice that the palms face out at the top and in at the bottom. When the arms are to the side, at shoulder height, the palms face down.

5. Perform the same exercise with the arms shoulder-width apart, overhead, palms facing forward (Photo 227). Press forward and down (wrists as well) (Photo 228), ending next to the hips, palms facing back (Photo 229). Return along the same line and press, press again.

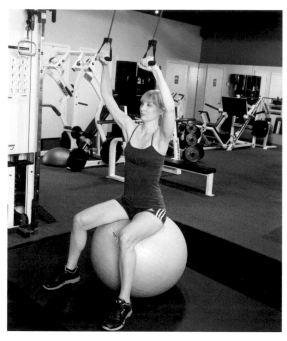

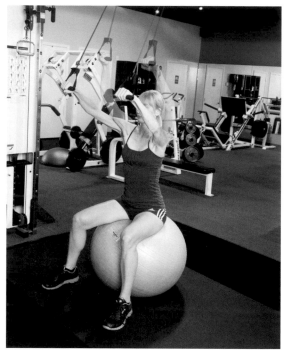

PHOTO 227

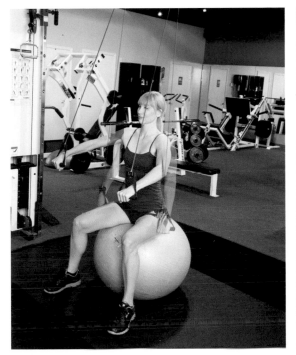

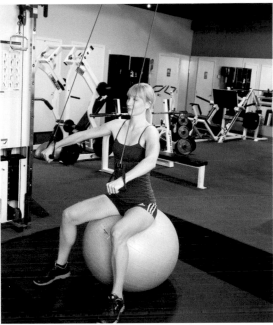

PHOTO 228

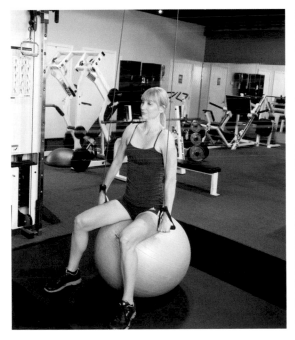

PHOTO 229

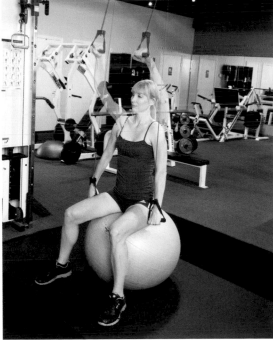

SEATED BAND TRICEPS PRESS

1. Use the same posture as step 5 in the previous exercise. With the forearms remaining vertical, pull your elbows down to your sides.

2. Lock your upper arms into your body and keep them immobile. The elbows are directly below the shoulders (Photo 230).

3. Using your grip, wrists and forearms, press forward and down until your arms are straight down at your side (Photo 231)

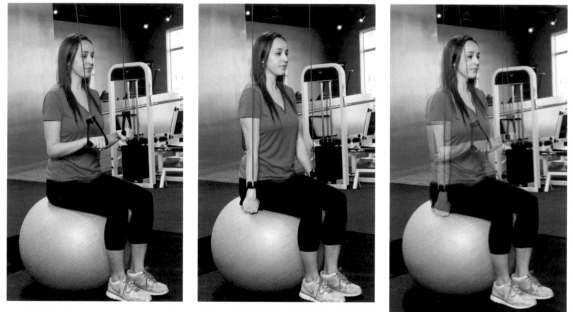

PHOTO 230   *PHOTO 231*

4. Without moving your elbows, bend and release. Do 10 to 20 reps.

A very safe way to work the muscles in the front of the shoulder assembly is to strengthen them isometrically, where they remain unmoving, yet vigorously employed in holding a true and solid form. Two examples come to mind that you might enjoy, which are not only of great benefit to the shoulders, but to your entire physique, provided you align yourself properly (most people don't).

The first, sometimes known as a type of **Plank**, is nothing more than a push-up without the pushing.

(NON) PUSH-UP

1. Assume a push-up position, arms roughly twice as wide as the shoulders.

2. Align the body as though standing up straight (see **Posture**, chapter II) (Photo 232).

Achieving this will require considerable thought and strength, as the body is nearly horizontal and supported on the hands and toes.

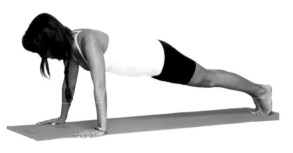

PHOTO 232

3. Don't do the push-up. Hold the position 20 seconds, 30 seconds and one full minute.

CHECKLIST

No dropped nose or chin jutting to the floor.

Pull out long through the back of the neck and align the crown of the head with the shoulders, butt and heels.

Don't round shoulders forward or lift them to the ears in pursuit of a jutting chin. Keep them secure, neither to the front or back, but instead firmly pressed down into your body.

Don't allow a hump in the middle or upper back. Stretch the torso out long and support strongly with your abs. (If your hump won't go away, check your chin and shoulders.)

Don't push your butt up in the air or drag the belly on the floor. The butt is tight; the lower belly's flat. The legs and feet are all the way together. The heels push out long to work the toes, feet and ankles, to stretch the knees and challenge the muscles along the top, bottom and sides of the entire structure.

Though strongly engaged, no muscles are gripped or frozen; no joints are locked. Full, deep, steady breathing keeps everything fluid and alive.

The healing potential of this exercise will become apparent in just a few days. Before long, you'll feel ready to add a little movement into the mix.

You can then start with very slight push-ups, bending the elbows just an inch or two. After a couple more days, add another inch, here and there, as you feel like it. Follow the 80% Rule and the potential for pain-free, full-range push-ups will soon again be yours.

HOVER

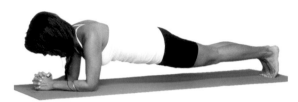

PHOTO 233

This exercise is identical to the **Non Push-Up** with two exceptions—it is performed with the arms bent, elbows and forearms flat on the ground and, rather than arms wide, the elbows are directly under the shoulders (Photo 233).

This makes a huge difference in what's required of the arms and shoulders, though most folks never seem to figure that out.

In a **Non Push-Up**, the elbows are open, the arms are extended. This position could not be maintained without force applied in the arms to control the elbow joints and keep the arms from buckling.

In the **Hover**, however, the arms have already buckled, and the forearms are flat on the ground. Therefore, there is no need to press into the floor to strengthen the elbows, nor to keep the upper-body elevated, neither with the fingers, the palms, the forearms, upper arms or shoulders. You see, the alignment of the bones of the upper arms makes it impossible for the upper torso to fall.

Think about it. The bones serve as vertical supports, like the legs of a table, right under your shoulders. They're not going anywhere. You could relax every muscle, letting your whole body slump into one gooey mass and still your shoulders would be hanging from those arm bones. Unless you're in the late stages of scurvy or your arms are about to be smacked by a big, angry man with a big, heavy club, your upper torso is not reaching the ground.

So, there's no need to push. No need to strain. Don't need no hump-backed whales, no chin-swept floors; don't need no high-butt bridges. Don't distract your body from all the good alignment work it could be doing.

Instead, use your extra strength to really settle those shoulders into the torso. Focus on lengthening your body into a straight stretch of railroad track, laying down a smooth ride all the way from the

Crown of Head Town through the Heels of Soul, passing through Shoulders Down, Flat Belly, Tight Butt, and Straight Knees along the way. It's a lovely journey when there's nothing else on your mind.

Pity of it is, most people automatically push down with their shoulders, even instructors. They don't even know they're doing it, it's just an instinctive response to a presumed gravitational necessity.

Such things as a misaligned **Hover** go a long way to teaching bad habits to the shoulders and the upper back. This can create a degree of ineptitude in all related muscles, especially the stabilizing faction of the rotator cuff. Get those guys mad at you, and you'll be working on this next one for a good few weeks.

STANDARD ROTATOR CUFF EXERCISE

This can be performed lying on the back, lying on one side, sitting or standing. Though the two isolated movements of the exercise, rotating the arm open and closed, remain the same throughout, the muscles work differently when the body lies at different angles, such as when it is horizontal as opposed to vertical. So, depending on the specifics of the injury, the victim may, for example, find more relief rotating the arm in one direction lying down, even though it feels better to move it in the other direction standing.

This same variable holds true for the hardware of choice. You will have different results depending on what you use—dumbbells, cables, resistance bands or internal muscular resistance (think moving isometrics—yes, I know, an oxymoron). Each different method creates different forces in the working shoulder, offering differing degrees of comfort and cohesion.

If the weight (and its accompanying gravitational pull) is in the hand, as with a dumbbell, the distribution of labor among the working muscles varies significantly from when the resistance is at a distance to the side, as with a cable. Even though both cables and bands use resistance from the side (in this exercise), their differing mechanics affect the way in which the muscles feel and respond to them. Each method creates a unique response in the working shoulder, and they are not all of equal benefit.

Remember, lots of muscles, little and big, are involved with the shoulders. It's not just the Rotator Cuff boys. The combination of body angle and choice of hardware have a direct impact on what you get out of this exercise and how quickly you get it.

For the execution of the exercise itself, standing with an exercise band will do nicely.

1. Stand strong, solid posture, feet hip-width apart.

2. Keep the elbow of the working arm close to or glued to the side of the body.
   Keep it there throughout. Bend the forearm to 90 degrees, palm facing in.

3. At an even pace, rotate the forearm open to the side, but only so far as it will go (approximately
   45 degrees) without causing the shoulder to move back, out of line with the body (Photo 234).

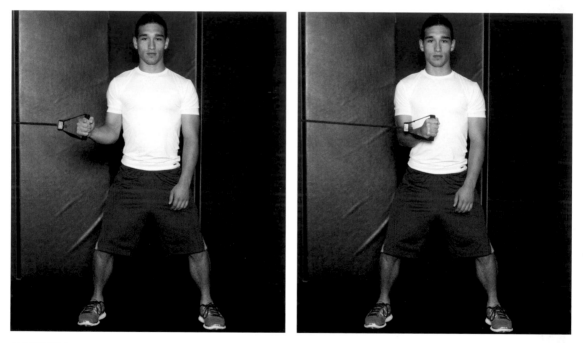

PHOTO 234   PHOTO 235

4. Having reached your outer limit, press the weight back in, towards your abs (Photo 235). Do not
   go so far that your elbow breaks contact with your side. Do 8 to 20 reps.

5. Change hands, so the band must be pulled open (Photo 236).

In this direction, the wrist can move as well. Roll it in as you pull, out as you open.

People often overdo this ROM in both directions, rotating a full 180 degrees. Going too far, in even
one direction, forces the working axis of the shoulder to shift, out of line, as it is turning, thereby
destabilizing the very joint you're trying to stabilize. From what I've seen, you'll do better keeping that
ROM closer to 90 degrees—45 in, 45 out—rather than 180.

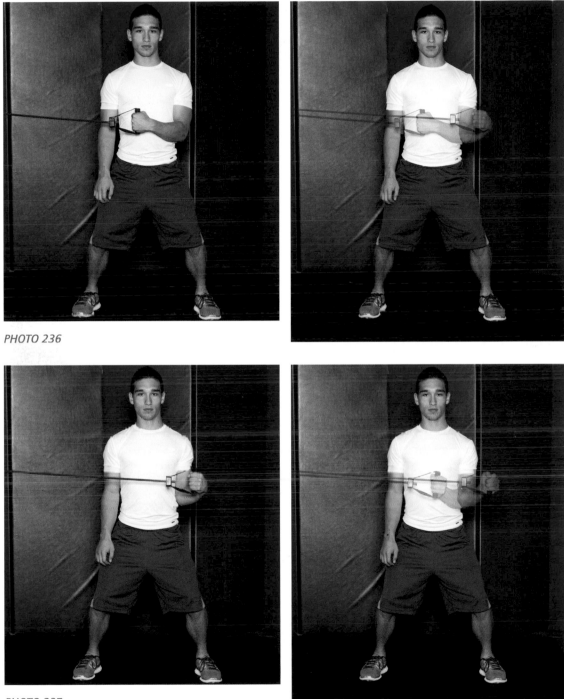

PHOTO 236

PHOTO 237

Keep a tight fist, a strong wrist, a strong forearm, elbow joint, upper arm and a shoulder properly placed (Photo 237).

THE TORSO

THE MIDDLE OF THE BACK

SYMPTOMS

A recurring zap, pinch, muscle soreness—or even numbness—in the middle of the back or to one side

ASSESSMENT

Injuries that appear in the middle of the back seem to come, almost exclusively, from one of two things: too much arching or too much sagging. Either can overtighten or overstretch the long muscles that support said (middle of the) back, not to mention heighten the opportunity for overcompressing or misaligning the vertebrae and discs of the spine in the area.

Created slowly and repetitively, through poor postural habits, or in the fouled misdeed of one fell moment, the progeny of such unnatural acts can be pesky, lingering and limiting.

WHAT TO DO

1. For an overstretched, rounded middle back:

Massage: Though relief can be had from acupressure, rollers and tennis balls (see **Neck and Shoulder Injuries**), the problem cannot be solved with massage alone. The muscles must be taught to take their places and do their jobs.

Stretches: Try the **Swiss Ball and Shoulder Rotation (Neck and Shoulder Injuries)**. More passively, try adding a small pillow behind your middle back while enjoying the **Couch-Assisted Shoulder Stretch, (Shoulder Injuries)**. Or leave the pillow there and just put your hands behind your head and relax completely.

Movement: Attention must be paid, as the area is strengthened, to improved postural and training habits. Being aware of what your structure is up to, whether active or passive, and knowing your limits when training is essential.

Exercises: Lat Pull-Downs, **Seated Upright Rows**, **Reverse Flies** (chapter VI), to wake up, strengthen and realign the posture of the middle back.

2. For an overarched, pinched middle back:

Massage: See step 1 previously.

Stretches: Do the following.

BALL-ASSISTED MIDDLE-BACK STRETCH

1. Standing, take a basketball, or a slightly larger ball, and place it against your solar plexus, immediately below your breastbone (Photo 238).
   This exercise can be also be done with a pillow or with muscular control alone.

2. Secure the ball within your arms, as though hugging it, and rotate your palms open, facing away from your body.

3. Drop your head slightly forward and press your elbows as far across your body as you can. This opens up the shoulder blades and increases the pressure of the ball against the body, making the middle back want to round.
   Allow your middle back to round into the stretch being offered by the pressure of the ball (Photo 239).

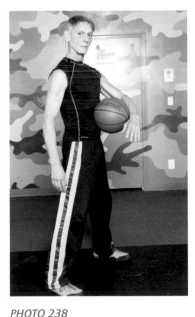

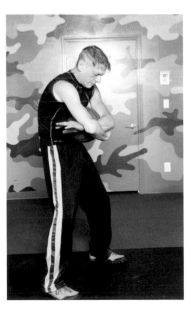

PHOTO 238   *PHOTO 239*

There is no need to raise the shoulders or to bend forward from the waist.

4. Breathe a sigh of relief.

A milder and more passive variation can be found by simply lying, chest down, on a Swiss ball, with the apex of the ball under the injured area. Relax completely, hang and breathe. The results, however, are not as dramatic.

Movement: As with a rounded, overstretched middle back, the solution lies in proper structure and support, which must be practiced consistently (see **Posture**, chapter II).

Exercises: Overarching tends to come from a lack of support in, at least, the upper abs, if not the entire belly and butt assembly. People with longer torsos, shorter women with larger breasts, and those whose parents were a little too intent on their kids standing up straight (seems to cause kids to overarch and stiffen) are often afflicted.

To set things right, your normal, strong, full-body workout will be fine. Just pay special attention to

(1) support in the (upper) abs, as described in **Posture** (chapter II), and in your entire rear assembly, from the back of your heels through the crown of your head; and

(2) the proper placement of the shoulders, which tend to pull too far back, in confluent aggravation, with the overarching of the middle back.

Severe straining of the middle back seems very rare. In fact, I've only seen it happen once, the day it happened to me.

Before it occurred, I would've thought that, since the legs and hips would remain uninjured, one could still get to one's feet and get around. What I didn't consider was that the muscles in the injured area, both in front and back, would become completely unresponsive.

If I had been less experienced, this incident would've scared the hell out of me. As it was, it took a while to calm my mind, and all my skill to keep from being bedridden for several days. I recall the play-by-play here for the sake of those more novitiate, to provide some light in an otherwise dark place:

Working hard in the gym, reaching high and fast into an extended arch, I felt the twinge when it happened, but it didn't seem that bad. I moved on to other exercises I thought would be safer, before spending a few hours, on my feet, training clients. By the time I finished, there was a moderate, steady pain in my middle back.

Then I drove the 45 minutes home. (If you really want an injury to take hold of you, sit down in one position, for a while, after it happens, and let it sink in.) By the time I arrived, I could hardly get out of my car. My body was functional from the waist down, and from the shoulders up, but there was a big, overstuffed suitcase of pain, loose in its straps, dragging behind me, where my middle back should have been.

Except for a modest control in my upper abs, I had no supportive connection between my shoulders and lower body. I managed getting out of my car by pulling with my arms, pushing from my hips, and balancing my ribcage, over my hips, as I moved.

Walking was something special. Picture a slender pedestal of two human legs, topped with a flat base, trying to balance an unsecured, top-heavy vase while making their way over uneven ground.

Funny to see, maybe, but not to be. Fortunately, I got inside my apartment just before my structure gave way.

I tried to resist as my body began to crumble into itself and my strength began to fail. I knew the deeper the hole the injury dug, the longer and harder my climb back out. And, once I'm contorted, muscles frozen, collapsed on the floor and unable to move, that hole gets pretty deep.

But my abs couldn't win the fight alone. And there was nothing to help. My mid-torso continued to contract, slowly and irrevocably, pulling my shoulders down and to the left, driven by a sharp, ever-increasing pain, which spread across my middle back and shot through the center of my body to the inside of my forward ribs, across and below my chest, paralyzing all it touched, attended notably by Messrs. Ache and Throb.

My legs weakened. My knees began to give way. I was doomed. I thought of the Mighty Kong, overcome by that last trail of bullets atop the Empire State Building, as I went down.

Yet, even as I fell, bent like a hook, I grasped out to reach a low table, tried to shift my upper body above it and take my weight into my arms and shoulders, to stop my knees from buckling. This caused my chest to freeze in agony, making it hard to breathe, but my arms and shoulders held, and I thought, for one brief moment, that I might be able, with one mighty push, to throw myself up straight again and get back to normal.

That didn't happen. My knees continued to drop. My head was falling low. My shoulders were being passed by.

My next line of defense was to try to take a knee and support my weight on my hips. Stop the fall. I slowly extended my bent thigh vertically below me and, supporting as I could with my arms, tried to lower my knee to the ground.

Immediately, the nerves in my middle back blew like an overloaded power line. One searing shock and every muscle below my shoulders failed—torso, hips, legs, feet. There was a desperate grab with my hands, a moment of helpless freefall, then I hit the floor hard.

I thumped down onto my right side, my muscles mid-torso contracting rigidly into a concrete mass, curling me up like a seahorse. I could feel them tightening—not a good sign.

I had to make a quick decision. Freezing up fast means freezing up hard, unless the process can be interrupted, but interrupting it is not always a good thing. On the other hand, if I didn't act immediately, I feared I might not be able to move from that spot on the floor for a couple of days. The situation was becoming dangerous.

Now, even when my lower back is at its worst, in an emergency, I believe I could manage to drag myself along by my arms. But here, as the lower parts of my big shoulder muscles were in the injured area, my middle back wasn't going to accept the stress of that heavy work.

I quickly realized that trying to push with my legs was also useless. Rather than making my whole-body move, pushing with my legs just made my lower body curl more into my middle back, prompting halting, incredulous gasps for air against the internal shock and awe that erupted through my ribcage.

I couldn't stay there much longer. The freeze was almost complete. But, I couldn't move forward; I couldn't move back.

That left rolling to the side. Rolling to the side meant getting onto my hands and knees. Maybe I could support myself on them, if I could get up on them to begin with.

I tested a press against the ground with my arm, gently tried to roll my upper body over, just an inch or so, to see how it felt. Pierced by a thousand points of pain, my muscles failed, and I was dropped back to the floor.

I knew what that meant. I'd been here before, many times. There was a barrier of pain, blinding, possibly broad, probably unsupportable, waiting, to be passed through, on my way up to my hands and knees.

That meant that, from my first push up from the side, until I reached the point of vertical support over my bones, I would have little or no ability to keep myself moving. I would have to create enough momentum with my initial push to propel me past any muscle failure this barrier might cause. And I had to move fast so that my body wouldn't have time to collapse if the nerves disconnected. If I could get up, I hoped enough of my neural control would return and my bones hold my weight, while I figured out my next step.

Trouble is, a hard initial push brings hard initial pain. And then, there's that infinitely long quarter second of otherworldly torment, that inquisitorial barrier, to pass through right after. I must admit, I felt a certain reluctance to begin, but it had to be done.

I managed to get my right hand under my right shoulder and my left palm on the floor, forward of my chest. Then I slowly squared my bent knees in front of my hips.

I took a long, deep breath, and pushed as hard as I could. For a moment I went interstellar, arcing skywards in a scorching blaze—"White Light, White Heat" (from the Velvet Underground's iconic album "Heroin"...What can I say? I've been around a long time.)

Then I was up! On top of my bones! And I could hold the position! And, glory of glories, the pain stabilized as soon as I had my balance. It was severe, but it was steady, not firing all over the place, no more fine shards of glass ripping through my torso at the speed of light. Nothing compared to riding the rocket that got me up there.

Crawling, on the other hand, was not so good. I felt stiff, unwieldy, unsure. My back wasn't happy.

And I wasn't going to be happy, just crawling around. Can't crawl to work in the morning. Not going to get much to eat crawling.

Somehow, I had to get back on my feet. Crawling my way toward the kitchen, I used the wall, leaning heavily against it, to claw my way up and eventually plop my torso, belly down, onto the kitchen counter. I breathed deeply, letting things relax, rallying my determination for what must come next.

Lying there, bent at the waist, was good. My feet still reached the floor, so I could raise my heels, as necessary, to ease the demise of my dromedary hump. Slow, deep breathing in that position went a long way to releasing the muscles involved.

After a couple of minutes, I placed my hands by my hips, palms down, on the edge of the counter, and performed the following. If you're ready for it, this position is helpful to virtually all the aches a back might tender.

PRESSING SHOULDERS, HANGING BODY

1. Stand against a counter or well-supported table that is at least as high as your waist. Bend your elbows, pull them back and place your palms on the top of the counter (Photo 240).
   Wrap your fingers (1) backward and down the front of the counter, or (2) forward across the countertop (personal preference). Keep your bent arms close to your body.

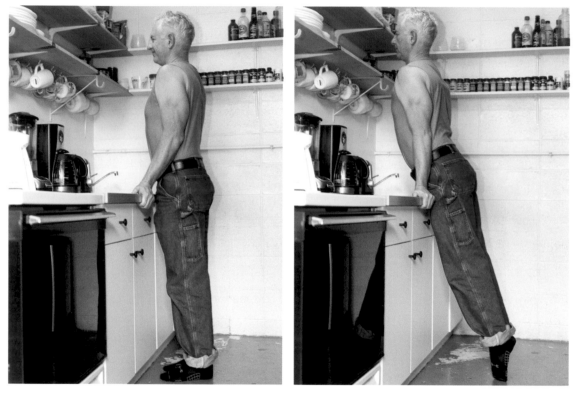

PHOTO 240   *PHOTO 241*

2. Pressing down with your shoulders and arms, lean slightly forward, until your body's weight rests securely over your hands.

3. Slowly straighten your elbows, taking care to relax everything hanging below the shoulders, with the possible exception of retaining some support with the legs, depending on how stressful the stretch is on the injury.

4. If it feels safe, straighten the arms all the way (Photo 241).
   This should bring the heels, if not the entire feet, off the floor. Hang freely from the shoulders and breathe deeply, letting the back relax and lengthen.

5. Never take this farther than you feel is safe (80% Rule). Stop when the time is right. Use as often as necessary.

Don't be surprised, when you come down onto your feet, if your body begins dropping back into the same injured posture from which you have just briefly escaped. Depending on the degree of injury, getting the muscles to relax and release is one thing, while their being capable of reassuming a full workload is something else.

To help mitigate any increased pain, collapse or attempted refreezing of the muscles once on your feet, don't just stand still. That'll work against you. Walk around a bit, lifting through the torso and breathing appropriately as you do. Try to walk in one direction, avoid a lot of turning. A lengthy straightaway can do wonders. Turns just interrupt the process. Walk at least two or three minutes if you can.

In my case, I wasn't surprised when my body dropped back into a hump when my weight was again on my feet. I was happy just to be standing. I seemed to have narrowly dodged a big bullet.

I immediately started walking, back and forth across my living room. I only lasted a few minutes before my muscles said stop, or else.

In increasing pain, I sat on my firm and supportive couch. To counter an attempted coup by back muscles loyal to refreezing, I lifted as tall as I could and leaned back, used my arms across the back of the couch to support. The process wasn't easy, but once there, I felt secure.

After a couple minutes of deep breathing to grow comfortable in this mild recline, I took a bead filled, tightly stuffed pillow (8 x 8 x 4) and placed it between my middle back and the back of the couch. Then I reached out, again back and wide, for the **Couch-Assisted Shoulder Stretch**, which I used to promote a mild arch in my middle back, as I breathed to relax the pain.

Once convinced my back wouldn't freeze up again, I reclined more deeply, with my back well supported, to let the trauma rest. Later, I began with a mild **Standing Hangover Bend and Stretch**, before trying the **Half Lotus Variation**, **Flutter-Bys** (all in chapter VIII), a few slow **Crossover Crunches** (chapter VI) and some low and easy **Pelvic Curls** (chapter II). After a couple of days, I was back to my regular workout, but I had to moderate some exercises for several weeks.

Though I didn't miss any work (and managed not to let my injury show in public), it took a couple of months to get a decent arch in my back again. The excessive pain lasted a good two or three weeks.

Even now, more than two years after the event, the right side of my middle back is still not quite the arching equal of my left. But, that could change any day.

INJURIES TO THE CHEST

The good news is that the breastbone (sternum) doesn't really move, so we're dealing primarily with strains and overuse here. The big chest muscles—the pectorals—reach out from the breastbone to the sides, working with the upper arm and shoulder assembly. Overstretching, a poor alignment of the arms and shoulders in stressful exercise, a too heavy load or too many reps, can all contribute to soreness in the chest muscles.

SYMPTOMS

1. Cramping and tightness throughout the pecs (not the Heart!)
   (Chest pain that can be touched with the fingers is on top of the ribs, and therefore musculoskeletal. Pain in the heart and lungs cannot be directly manipulated.)

2. A finger's width of pain, steady or fluttering, reaching across one, or both, sides of the chest; pain that seems to appear in just one spot out to the side or in at the breastbone, or a combination of these two. (These symptoms may only appear in certain postures.)

3. Soreness or tightness particularly at the upper outside corners of the chest, right where they join the shoulders

ASSESSMENT

1. If it's mild, no big deal. You had a good workout. If it really hurts, you've pushed too much weight too many times.

2. This sort of thing is usually the result of overstretch or poor form, as with **Chest Flies**, **Bench Press** (both in chapter VI), or **Push-Ups**, or overuse in any of these. As well, with the finely-tuned requirements of an exercise like push-ups on the fingertips, anything in the structure—a finger, the wrist, a muscle in the arm or shoulder—needs only falter for a moment to cause a strain farther up the line, in this case, in a finger's width of the pecs, or in the muscles, between the ribs, that lie beneath them.

3. This area is usually sore when it has been overworked (see 1). However, it can also be strained from overstretching.

WHAT TO DO

Massage: Acupressure is your friend.

1. Use all your fingers and play those chest muscles like castanets, drumming the fingers strongly across, working primarily from the breastbone out to the sides.

2. Requires a more specific approach. Using one or two fingers, start where you feel the pain, with steady, motionless pressure, then drum your way out to either end, applying more, or more sustained, pressure where needed. You may find tender spots at the breastbone that benefit from extra attention.

3. Same as 1, but some steady, unmoving pressure may be helpful as well.

Stretches: For all three, **Shoulder Rotation and ROM** (chapter II), **Swiss Ball and Shoulder Rotation** and **Couch-Assisted Shoulder Stretch**. Work ROM to stretch symptoms **1** and **3**, and to guide symptom **2** to safely and healthfully rejoin the team. If these are all right, you can move on to **Arm Swings** (chapter VIII).

Movement: For all three, avoid oversqueezing the chest (inwardly), or overstretching, out and back, to the sides.

Exercises: To help equalize the area, the **Lat Pull-Downs**, **Seated Upright Rows** and **Reverse Flies** (chapter VI) will all help. Otherwise, your regular upper-body workout, reducing the weight, reps and ROM as necessary.

OVERWORKING THE ABS

As with the chest, strains and overuse are the prime causes of pain in the abs and the muscles to either side of them (primarily, the *obliques*).

SYMPTOMS

1. Cramping, as with the flu or food poisoning

2. Steady or fluttering pain, localized or linear, in normal posture or when arching or twisting, anywhere from the lower ribs down to the pubic bone

ASSESSMENT

1. If it's not the flu or food poisoning, most likely you overdid your ab workout and the muscles, not your insides, are the source of the pain.

2. Localized pain, at the ribs or along the side of the belly, might suggest a strain in a tendon, where a linear pain in the body of the muscle would suggest a strain of (a bundle of) muscle fibers within the muscle itself. Remember, also, there is a line of interconnective tissue down the middle of the abs and there are tendon-type bands that reach across the abs, creating the six-pack divisions that can be strained.

WHAT TO DO

Massage:

1. As with **Injuries to the Chest**, symptoms **1** and **3**, "Play, magic fingers!" Drums along the Mohawk of your belly and ease that cramping pain. You may have to go a little lighter than on the chest, as you wouldn't want to disturb the comfort of all those internal organs just underneath.

2. Approach as with injuries to the chest, symptom **2**.

Stretches: For symptom **1**, anything that lifts and lengthens the abs will do the trick. For instance, lie prone on the floor and place your arms on the floor above your head, slightly wider than your shoulders. Breathe deeply.

You might also try the following.

DOOR FRAME STRETCH

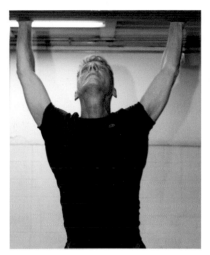

1. Stand before a doorway, feet facing forward. Place your arms high and wide against the frame.

2. Supporting with your arms, lean forward and up, lifting through the chest (lift your head to give your chest room to rise) (Photo 242).

Squeeze your stretching abs.

More actively, try the **Swiss Ball and Shoulder Rotation**, paying special attention to your arching back and stretching abs.

PHOTO 242

For symptom **2**, stretching the injury directly may not feel too good, and you may have to curtail your ROM in the injured area for a few days. (If the injury is more to one side, be sure to curtail the other side's activities to the same degree, as not to cause an imbalance in your healing structure.) If you attempt any direct stretch of the injury, begin slowly and gently, as with lying prone and slowly taking the arms overhead to the floor.

You may find it easier to stretch a vertical ab injury with an appropriately angled, slightly arched lean to the side, either standing or lying down (see **All of Your Twist**, chapter VIII). As the focus of this stretch is not directly along the line of the injury, it may not be as stressful to it. Of course, if the injury is a twisting one, you may want to reverse this suggestion.

Movement:
1. Don't slouch. Keep your torso lifted and long. The lower you collapse your chest toward your hips, the more opportunity for the abs to contract and cramp. Don't let your belly hang out, either. It could easily make it hurt more and will definitely work against all the work you overdid to get it in shape.

2. Determine when it hurts the most and, if necessary, avoid such postures or movements to the degree that they work against your recovery.

Exercises: With both symptoms, continue with your regular routine, modified, of course to not overwork the injury (80% Rule, please). If some exercises are out of the question, perhaps there are healthful alternatives. The injured area doesn't have to be the main focus of the exercise. It may get all the work it can handle as an assistant.

TWISTING INJURIES

Twisting injuries come from, and are treated the same as, injuries to the abs, sides, middle and lower-back. As the first three are already discussed, let's get on to the motherload.

THE LOWER BACK

I believe the percentage of people who suffer lower-back injury or chronic pain is considerably higher than that of any other structural malady dealt with in this book. Everyone knows someone who displays the telltale signs of discomfort, even if they don't talk about it. Whether along the spine, or to one or both sides along the top of the hips, whether localized and dull or firing taser-blasts through the hips and down the legs, the inhibition of movement and preoccupation of mind that trouble those misfortunate, can be a strong detractor to one's quality of life.

Thing is, I don't believe it's necessary, for most of those who suffer, and it doesn't seem that hard to fix. It's just a matter of knowing how and fixing it. Even those who have good reason to suffer, from congenital defects (as with my lower spine), or serious injury and surgical repair, can do a lot, in most cases, to minimize their pain and physical limitation.

ASSESSMENT

Clearly, if there is pain, nerves are being affected. The question is whether these affectations are caused directly or secondarily.

1. Directly, nerves can be compressed as they exit the spine, stressed by overtight muscles along their routes and pinched by the joints between the vertebrae and others through which they pass.

2. Secondarily, soft tissue injuries—to ligaments, tendons and muscles—through misuse, overuse and plain old accident can cause nerves to scream equally loudly.

Most lower-back problems involve a combination of both. Though each different injury may vary in degree, location and maleficent sensation, the approach to discovery and recovery is largely the same. Injuries to this part of the body rarely, if ever, occur in isolation, but rather are always connected to larger structural inequities. Therefore, to ensure a comprehensive recovery, a comprehensive approach is best taken.

The goal is fourfold:

1. Open up the vertebrae of the spine and allow the discs to realign and reexpand into their appropriate positions, taking any undue pressure off the nerves.

2. Relax any tight or knotted muscles and bring them into an harmonious and flexible balance with their neighbors.

3. Relieve and retrain any strained muscles or tendons.

4. Bring all of the above into a healthful, unified whole.

To do any less would be to treat the symptom, not the source. As with the neck and shoulder assembly, the area is complexly integrated. No pain is an island. You can be sure, if one thing's wrong, it's got friends.

WHAT TO DO

Massage: Depending on the injury, massage can prove very useful, especially if the root cause is muscular. However, unless you've been down that road before and know the lay of the land, have the caregiver start off very easy, and don't be shy about speaking up along the way.

Chiropractics and acupuncture may be helpful as well. Unfortunately, for my spinal situation, none of these have succeeded in giving any more than very limited, very temporary relief.

Stretches and Exercises: These depend on the degree to which your injury inhibits your ability. I have defined four basic categories:

1. If you are stiff and sore, but you can work, any stretches and exercises that feel helpful are allowed. I would suggest the stretches in chapter VIII, in order of appearance, to warm the body up and open up the back and hips. After that, the supine ab and hip exercises, from chapter VI, modified as necessary, to safely strengthen the core and its environs.

2. If you can't move very well, but you can sit in a chair (and for minimum daily maintenance), try the **Seated Hangover Stretch**.

3. If you can't yet sit, but you can struggle to your feet, try **Pressing Shoulders**, **Hanging Body**. Depending on how secure you feel after that, you can try the **Wall-Supported Hangover Stretch**. After these, you might be able to do some **Walking**.

4. If you have been bedridden and are just beginning to crawl, see **Reverse Sitting**.

SEATED HANGOVER STRETCH

Happily, this is a very easy and, basically, passive (believe it or not!) stretch, for beginning work on any lower-back problem, and it offers quick relief. It is the "at least" of all the lower-back work I recommend. If you will do nothing else to ease your back and hip pain, at least do this. I can't think of anyone who hasn't felt a little better the first time they tried it and, when used regularly, improved consistently over days and weeks, with full benefits realized within a few months.

I have given this stretch to hundreds of people over the years, and I have heard nothing but good things in return. To my knowledge, no one has ever been injured in its application.

The worst I have seen comes from the occasional chronic sufferer who has already tried, and found wanting, any number of professionally suggested solutions for their pain. Some such people appear to have developed a pointed skepticism to anything new that might come down the pike, and this seems to inhibit their ability to give a different process an honest shot. Said skepticism tends to preoccupy their minds (and their mouths) throughout the exercise, preventing any real relaxation.

The usual response, after such moderate attempts, is, "Yeah, that's nice," sometimes delivered with a dash of condescension, presumably to my deluded belief that something so simple could relieve their chronic pain.

I have occasionally wondered if such responses are due purely to an intellectual dismissal of the method, or if, maybe, some folks just don't want to lose an old friend, or an old excuse, no matter how much of a pain in the back it may be. Unfortunately, as these unhappy few will never seriously access this stretch, they will never know its bountiful rewards.

The one or two of these people I run across regularly, continue to struggle with lower-back pain, and continue to be dismissive of this method they will not honestly try.

"Y'see, Slim, you got this horse and then there's this water..."

As the name of the stretch suggests, in broad terms, one sits down and hangs over. Of course, if you're in a lot of pain, this relief must be sipped on, not gulped. Simply sitting down and trying to hang forward won't do you much good. Such a big movement from the whole torso all at once can shock the heck out of a bad injury and set your recovery back days or weeks. Some have found this approach too painful, on the first try, to ever want to attempt the stretch itself again and have removed it from their therapeutic possibilities.

Which is a pity because, when properly instructed, and gently employed, this stretch can be a life changer. When approached in the "from the top down, one vertebra at a time" method described next, starting with nothing more than a slow drop of the chin, anyone who can sit up can find surprising relief.

1. Sit on a firm bench or chair of a height that allows your thighs to remain parallel to the floor. Sit forward near the edge, but not so far that your legs will take the weight when you lean forward with your torso (Photo 243).

Your weight should remain solidly in your hips, on the seat, throughout this maneuver.

If you're in a lot of pain, it may be necessary to support your back externally to safely sit up straight. In this case, sit all the way back in the seat and support against the back of the chair. Though the stretch will be somewhat diminished, safety first!

Feet face forward, slightly more than hip-width apart, wide enough for the shoulders to pass between the knees, which are bent to 90 degrees, directly over the feet, in alignment with the toes and hips. Hands rest, or help support, on the thighs.

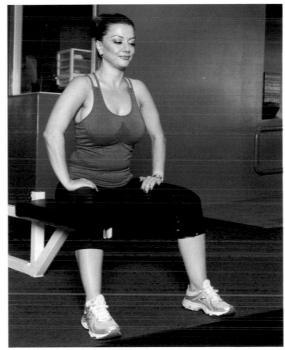

2. Sit tall. Lift through the back of the neck and *PHOTO 243* the top of the head. Inhale deeply.

3. Supporting with your belly, as you exhale, slowly take your chin forward and down, toward your chest. Keep the back of the neck stretching long. If you are really debilitated, this may be as far as you will want to go. You'll know by the way it feels. It's a pain of recovery sort of thing, very obvious when you hit that first spot. You may not reach your chest. You may not go very far at all.

4. If, however, you're doing all right, as the head reaches its full forward pitch, follow with the torso, rolling it forward and down, one vertebra at a time, taking the head and shoulders down between the knees. Keep your weight firmly in your hips on the bench, support with your belly.

Think out and away from the hips with the body, not just straight down. Optimize the length of the entire spine.

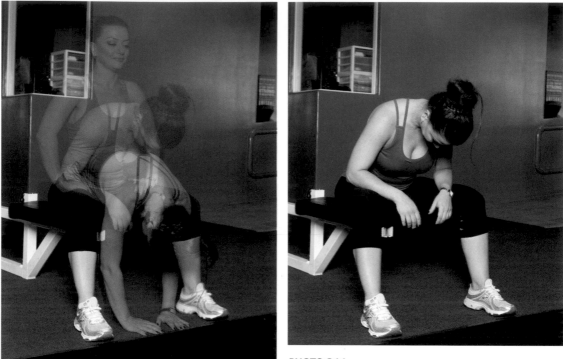

PHOTO 244

If your back is weak, or this is painful but doable (within the 80% Rule), use your hands, on your thighs, to take the extra weight as you move. Once you are low enough, the forearms will reach the thighs and take over for the hands (Photo 244).

5. Roll down as far as feels helpful. As the shoulders pass between the thighs, extend the hands to the floor. There, they and the arms may completely relax or be used for support (Photo 245).

Optimally, the torso will hang at full length, though it may need continual auxiliary support from the hands and arms to do so. When your support structure is badly compromised, even a split second without such steady assistance can be expensive. To keep your support more consistent, when making the transition from the forearms on the thighs to the hands on the floor, a couple of books stacked between the feet will make an easier reach for the hands than the floor.

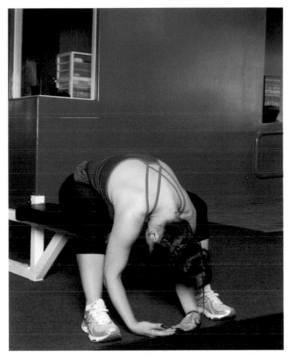

6. Once at your hanging limit, whether it be no more that a half-inch drop of your chin or your whole torso melting below your hips, remain there and breathe. And I mean, **Breathe!** (See **Deep Breathing**, **Neck and Shoulder Injuries**). Inhale deeply, from the lower back

PHOTO 245

up; exhale smoothly, from the head and shoulders down. The more you relax, the better it works. If you're completely relaxed, each inhale will cause a visible rise in your torso while, with each exhale, your head will drop a few millimeters lower to the ground. But, it won't happen if you're trying.

You might also enjoy placing the hands across the back of the shoulders while you're hanging (Photo 246).

Great for the neck and shoulders, though more stressful on the lower back.

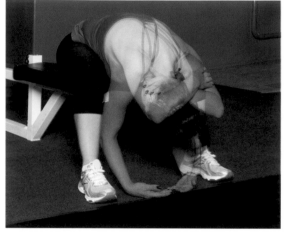 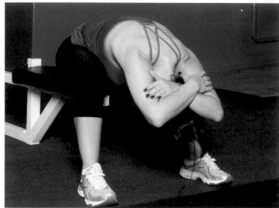

PHOTO 246

However you hang, don't try to stretch, don't think about other things. Just forget the world and breathe.

7. After about a minute, take a deep breath, then exhale as you roll your body up, one vertebra at a time, supporting with your belly, from the hips through the head, which is the last to unfurl.

8. Remain sitting tall and draw the legs and feet together until they are hip-width apart. Keep one foot solidly on the floor, maintaining the hip-knee-toe alignment. Lift the other, open the hip and place the ankle, above its bony bump, across the supporting thigh, in the softer recess immediately above the knee (Photo 247).

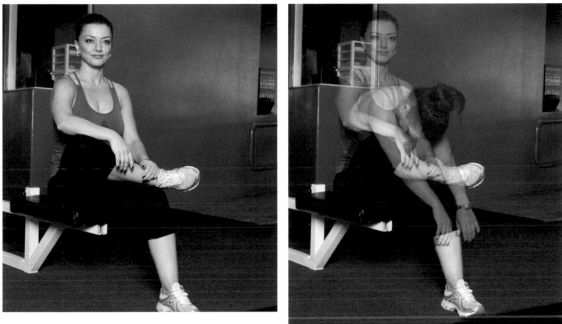

PHOTO 247

If your pain is in one hip or one side of your back, start with the opposite leg.

9. Repeat steps 2 through 7 (Photo 248), working both sides.

Three times a day, folks, that's all it takes. Nine minutes out of your life each day. Even if you don't address any deeper problems of structure and support, even if you do no regular exercise, when used daily, this stretch brings relief. I'm not saying it's all you should do, but it does comprise the most effective "at least" that I know.

So, make yourself happy. If, or once, you can work harder than this, other stretches and exercises become available (see previous **What to Do** section). These will vary, in order of appearance and degree of accessibility, as necessary, depending on your injury's specifics.

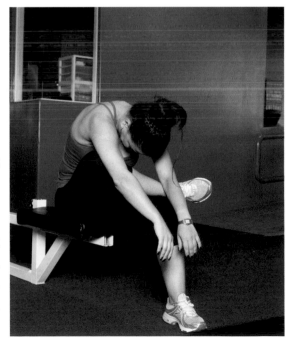

PHOTO 248

WALL-SUPPORTED HANGOVER STRETCH

1. Standing as best you can, rest your butt and your back, if possible, against a wall. Take the feet out from the wall a foot or so, hip-width apart, and bend your knees to about 30 degrees, until supporting your weight against the wall feels as close to comfortable as it's going to get.

2. With your hands supported on your thighs (Photo 249), follow steps 3 through 7 for the **Seated Hangover Stretch**.

If your hands on your thighs don't give enough support as you lean forward, place the back of a chair in front of yourself and hold onto it as you roll down. Remember the 80% Rule!

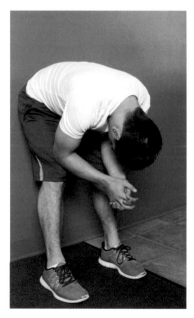 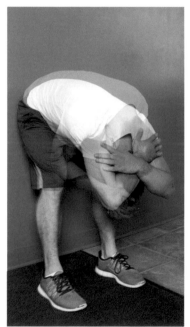 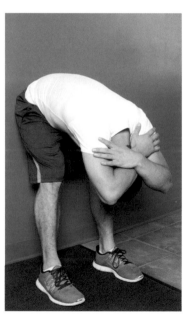

PHOTO 249   PHOTO 250

If you feel all right, well then. (Photo 250)

WALKING

Walking, with complete focus on support and alignment, really helps a body straighten out when it's been compromised. You've got to be ready for it, though. If you can stand entirely on your feet, hands free, and maintain some degree of erectitude through your torso, you can give it a shot.

Ideally, this walking would be done on a completely flat and level surface, where one could go at least 50 or 60 feet without having to turn (turning isn't helpful). Moving straight ahead, at a decent pace, the locked and frozen muscles of the injured area start to loosen up and realign in a more healthful design (don't forget to breathe).

I have walked as long as 20 minutes before reaching what felt like the optimum posture available to my injured back at the time. In most such cases, to find enough straight ahead walking space, I had to venture outside, where every little bump in the sidewalk, every degree of slant in the pavement, every miniscule incline and decline, every step off the curb, were painfully prominent.

Nevertheless, I walked that crooked mile, and every now and then, as I walked, some previously obstinate contortion in my lower trunk would soften and shift back into a more natural position. After a few days, my torso would straighten out within minutes of beginning my walk. Shortly thereafter, I could align myself properly within moments of standing.

A helpful addition to walking, which I discovered accidentally one day, is to carry weight in your hands while walking. I was three or four days into getting on my feet after six weeks unable to do so, and my girlfriend was leaving for Europe. Still quite twisted, still in a lot of pain, I determined to carry her luggage out to the corner and hail her a cab.

To my great surprise, carrying her bags, with relatively equal weight in both hands, straightened me out in a hurry. It was hard to pick them up, and the pain increased initially from their weight, but, within moments of walking, I felt the benefit: I was suddenly more solid, more in control, more vertical than I had any reason to hope for.

After that, whenever I was in recovery for my lower back, as soon as I could handle it, I would begin walking with weights in my hands. It speeds up the process.

In the course of your own recovery, once you feel able, add appropriate stretches and exercises to your improving routine (see previous **What to Do** section).

REVERSE SITTING

When my back has been severely injured, this is the first thing I try to accomplish, once I am no longer bedridden and finally able to crawl (in my worst case so far, it took four days before I could crawl with relative safety). I'm not saying it isn't difficult and doesn't hurt like hell to get there, but laying in bed doesn't feel much better and, after a point, is no longer effective for a strong and speedy recovery. The softness of a bed can actually become a detriment, while a firm floor, as used in **Reverse Sitting**, becomes an asset (if the floor is too hard, put down a towel or firm mat).

1. Place an easily moveable chair within easy reach. Lay on your side, on the floor, with your knees bent up toward your chest, as in a mild fetal position (Photo 251). (If you're really hurting getting to this position, achieve your fetal posture on your hands and knees, then try to gently and thoughtfully roll down onto one side.)

2. Pull the nearest front leg of the chair up behind you, bringing the outside front corner of the seat to the back of your hips, so that the seat is facing lengthwise up the back of the torso (Photo 251).

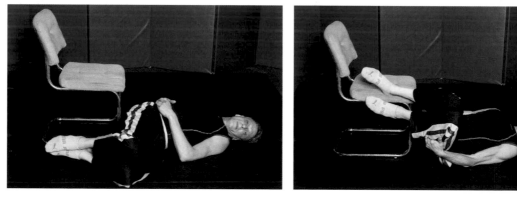

PHOTO 251   PHOTO 252

The idea is that when you roll onto your back, you will line up with the chair, with the front of its seat vertically above your hips.

3. Grab your upper calf, just below the knee, with your upper hand. Hold it firmly into the chest. Press your lower hand and arm into the floor for support. Using only the upper arm, rotate the upper thigh open to the side (vertically) toward the chair's seat.

4. As your back rotates toward the floor and the lower thigh begins to lift, switch the lower hand to the lower calf, just below the knee (Photo 252).

Use your upper-body strength to both rotate the legs vertically and, at the same time, mitigate the stress and pain in the lower back as you move (Photo 253).

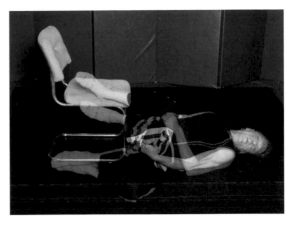

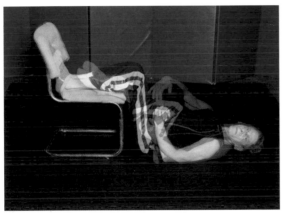

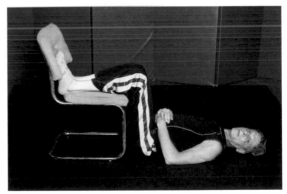

PHOTO 253

5. As your back comes flat to the floor, place your calves in the chair's seat (Photo 254).

The seat of the chair should be high enough to firmly support the entire calves, without lifting the lower back, in any way, from the floor. Thighs should be vertical, hips and knees bent to 90 degrees.

PHOTO 254

6. Rest in this position, as much as you like. A pillow may be placed under the head, but don't let your chin pop up and the back of your neck contract. Lengthen your entire spine, squeeze your belly a bit, if it's not too painful, and work on your breathing. Wait a day or two before trying to get things moving.

When, after that day or two, you feel you are capable, lie supine with knees bent and feet on the floor. Very gently, try the low **Pelvic Curls** (chapter II). Keep in mind, your low **Pelvic Curls** might go no farther than a mild squeeze of the buttocks and belly, with little or no actual curling taking place. Your butt may not even leave the floor.

If this feels all right, you might try **Single-Knee Lifts.**

SINGLE-KNEE LIFTS

1. Lie supine on the floor, knees vertical, bent to 90 degrees, feet supported on the floor. The lower-back is flat on the floor (Photo 255).
   Hands are at the sides, palms down.

2. Squeeze your belly and lift one knee up and in toward the torso (Photo 256).

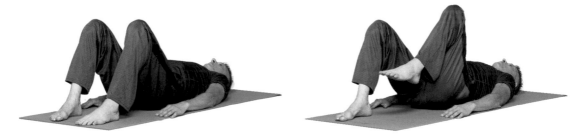

PHOTO 255   PHOTO 256

Depending on your injured ability (the 80% Rule), this action might cause the knee to rise no more than a fraction of an inch. Remember, it's not about how far it goes, it's about activating the area to the extent that is healing and helpful, which, at first, may be a very minor extent indeed, with very few repetitions involved.

3. Place it back down. If this is too tough, press your arms and palms into the ground for extra support as it lowers. If that's not enough, grab the thigh with your hands and use your upper-body strength to help lower it safely. If that's still too hard, place books under the feet to shorten the movement, decrease the angle and ease the pain. (The highest stress on the lower back occurs when the feet first lift from the floor and just before they reach it coming down again.)

4. Once the first foot is firmly on the floor again, try the other leg. The number of reps is case specific.

From here, very small Crunches can be attempted, followed by severely abridged **Single-Leg Lifts** (chapter VI), starting with the leg vertical and lowering no more than 45 degrees. If that works out, mild **Crossover Crunches** (also chapter VI) could follow, and then, perhaps, an attempt at higher **Pelvic Curls** (chapter II).

Working on this sequence of movements would be plenty for the first day or two. When resting, continue to employ **Reverse Sitting** if useful.

Though even that little bit of movement will probably make you quite sore the next day, don't take a day off, unless you think you've hurt yourself again. Rather, continue what you've started and safely add to the sequence.

As soon as you can stand, go on to **Pressing Shoulders**, **Hanging Body**, the **Wall-Supported Hangover Stretch** and **Walking**. Once you can sit again, add the **Seated Hangover Stretch**. Try, every day or two, to incorporate more and more of the stretches and exercises described here, in the order given, as possible and moderated as necessary, into your therapy. First those seated and supine, geared to the hips and trunk, then sprinkle in the easier standing ones. Eventually the harder stuff can be added, as you proceed down the road to your fullest possible recovery.

Along the way, I would use every tool at my disposal—heat, ice, sleep, tennis balls, anything I could think of, if it seemed it might help. Of course, I would constantly be guided by the three pillars of any solid recovery—Understanding, Patience and Consistency.

Movement: As your lower back heals, keep in mind that, though most movements may feel fine, other than, perhaps, some stiffness, the particular movement or posture that caused your trouble will remain more sensitive to both pain and reinjury for some time. One wrong move could put you right back where you started. Teach your body well so that you won't have to think before it will respond to protect you from that one false move.

THE HIPS AND BUTTOCKS

Being as closely related as they are to the lower-back assembly, recovery from most injuries to the hips and buttocks begin with the same approaches, stretches and exercises that work for the lower back. Though these may prove adequate, there are a few more to be considered, whether for continued therapy or general healthful maintenance.

SYMPTOMS (THE PAIN CAN BE SHARP, DULL, OR THROBBING)

1. Pain along the ridge of one or both hips

2. Pain running from the hips or buttocks down into the back of the legs

3. Pain in the hips or buttocks when the knees or legs are rotated or stretched open to the sides

4. Pain in the hip sockets (underneath the bottom of the buttocks), possibly extending down the outside of the legs or up into the cheeks and hips

ASSESSMENT

1. An injury of this type may be located in the lower back or in the hip. The symptoms are very similar for both, as are the remedies.

2. This could occur from either the lower back, the hip sockets, the muscles on the back of the thigh, or some combination of these.

3. This problem will be found in the rotator muscles of the buttocks, often compounded by tight (when rotated open) or imbalanced inner thighs.

4. This particular sensation is caused, in every case I've seen so far, by the outside of the legs taking a disproportionate share of the load on a regular basis, while the inner thighs (especially) and the inner calves, do less than they should.

WHAT TO DO

Massage: This can be helpful for all these symptoms, though you may have to look around to identify all the muscles involved. For instance, symptom **4** often comes with issues in the hip rotators (in the cheeks of your backside), but you never feel pain in them until you go exploring.

What does very nicely, especially to mitigate the pain that comes from sitting for lengths of time, is a tennis ball or two. Placed appropriately, these can make all the difference in comfort and continuing relief.

Stretches:

1. In most cases, the **Seated Hangover Stretch** will help, particularly steps 8 and 9. If, however, the pain is on the side of the body, and not in the back, **All of Your Twist** and **Weather Vanes** (chapter VIII) may do you better. Keep in mind, though, **Weather Vanes** are best done when the body has already been warmed up.

   Also helpful should be the **Standing Bend and Stretch**, the **Half Lotus Variation**, **Flutter-Bys** and **Knees to the Chest** (chapter VIII).

2. Everything from symptom **1**. **Leg Swings** and the **Reclining Single-Leg Stretch** (chapter VIII) should help as well.

   In addition, there is a **Standing Single-Leg Stretch**, which, when done right, often surprises the newcomer with its bounteous rewards. It can be of particular use in cases such as this.

STANDING SINGLE-LEG STRETCH

One leg is lifted and extended onto a supporting surface, such as a table, the back of a couch or a heavy and immoveable chair. In a gym, one may find a railing, a platform of the right height, a ballet bar or some part of an exercise machine.

A **Preacher Curl bench**—used here—works very well, as the height can be adjusted to the flexibility of the user and it is well padded. (Someone really tight may need a surface no higher than the knees to start.) If you use an unpadded railing, place a folded towel between it and the calf.

Whatever is used must be thoroughly stable, particularly for those stiffer and new to this. It is also desirable to have something stable to hold onto, with at least one hand, for extra support and stability, as the body balances on one foot throughout the stretch.

1. Standing, face the bench at a 45-degree angle, heels together, toes open (knees rotated open). Use your inside hand to support, if necessary, elbow slightly forward of the body so that your shoulder remains in its proper alignment and does not rotate forward.

2. Lift your outside leg and stretch it forward, resting the lower calf, still rotated open, on the platform (Photo 257).

Flex your foot and engage the muscles through the hip.

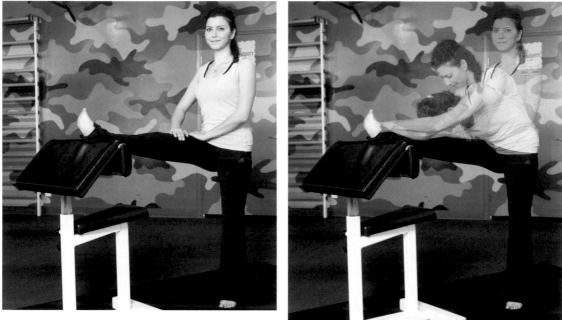

PHOTO 257

3. Engage and stretch your supporting leg. Lift tall through the body and slowly drop forward, head first, as you exhale. Once at your extension, flex and point the foot and toes a couple of times (Photo 258).

4. Rotate the working leg in and flex and point (Photo 259).

5. Now rotate the (straight and strong) standing leg, from knee and foot open to the side, to knee and foot facing forward. As you do, rotate the working leg open. Flex and point a couple of times, finishing in a point.

6. Again rotate the working leg to vertical alignment. Flex and point a yet again.

7. When you're ready, roll the body up, bring the leg down, change sides and work the other leg in similar fashion.

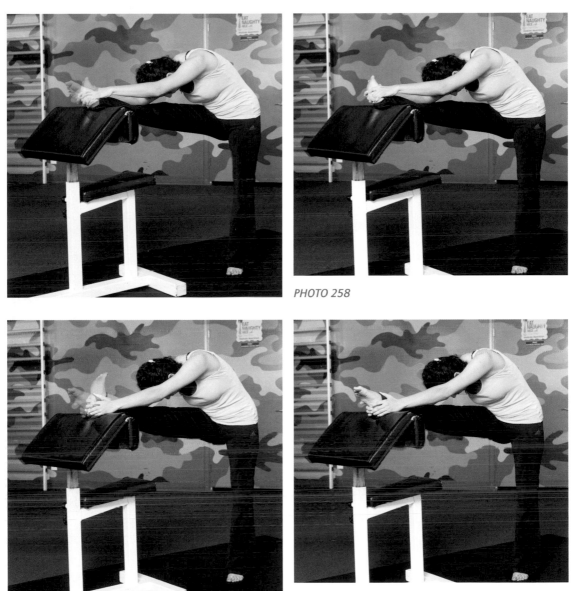

PHOTO 258

PHOTO 259

For symptom **3**, everything from symptoms **1** and **2** is useful. In addition, do the **Legs Wide** stretches (chapter VIII), but not until you're warm.

There is one more stretch, as well, which has an easier, more passive version, if you're not warmed up, or a more challenging one for the end of your workout. Though it has similarities to the **One-Leg Wide** version of **Legs Wide** stretches (chapter VIII), which are performed sitting on the floor, pay attention to the differences, for these are what alter the effect on the working areas.

SEATED SINGLE-HIP STRETCH

(This is the easy one.)

1. Straddle a bench (preferably padded). Sit near one end, facing the other end. Place one bent leg on the bench. Open the knee to the side and rest the calf across the bench, anchored by the ankle's bony bump so that the foot hangs free. The calf should cross the midline of the body about halfway between the ankle and the knee (Photo 260).

Keep the supporting foot firmly on the floor, knee bent to approximately 90 degrees, hip, foot and toes aligned.

2. Extend the working knee (the one turned open on the bench) to an angle about three-quarters straight.

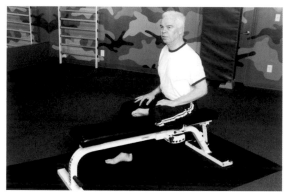

PHOTO 260

3. Sit tall, take a deep breath and roll the body forward and down, arms reaching, hands leading along the bench (keep those shoulders down). Go as far as you can, relax the stretched arms and hands at their extension, stay there and breathe a while.

4. When you're ready, roll the body up as you exhale.

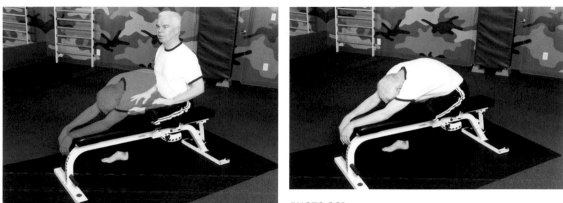

PHOTO 261

5. Repeat step 3 with the working knee at a more acute angle, with the heel of the working foot flush against the inside of the (90-degree bent) supporting knee.

6. Repeat step 3 with the working foot drawn all the way into the hips, as with the lower foot in the **Half Lotus Variation** (chapter VIII) (Photo 261).

7. Change sides.

STANDING SINGLE-HIP STRETCH

(This is the harder one.)

1. Find a supporting surface of the right height for the working leg (see **Standing Single-Leg Stretch**). Face the surface, standing tall, heels together, toes open.

2. Hold on with the hands, as needed, to stabilize. Bring one knee up, turn it open and place the length of the calf, from the knee to the ankle, across the surface (Photo 262).

Stand close enough that the working knee always remains at an acute angle without having to lean forward from the hips.

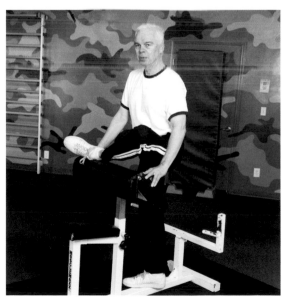

PHOTO 262

3. Take a deep breath and roll forward and down, with the torso, on the exhale (Photo 263).
   Keep the hips aligned above the standing leg and try to keep the standing leg straight. Squeeze
   your belly and keep your shoulders down.

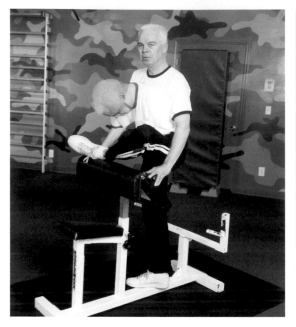

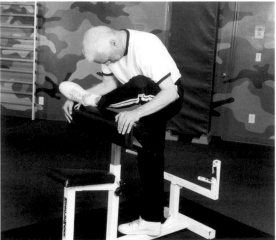

PHOTO 263

4. Make sure the working leg is well supported, form the knee through the ankle, at all times.

5. When you're ready, roll up on an exhale, bring the leg down, and begin to the other side.

Symptom **4**. Everything from symptoms **1**, **2** and **3**, with these considerations:

Passively, the **Seated Hangover Stretch**, the second part, with one ankle across the opposite knee,
and both the seated and standing **Single-Hip Stretch** will be of special help. Actively, the **Half Lotus
Variation** and the **Standing Bend and Stretch** (chapter VIII) especially bringing the legs together
when the toes are turned open, might hit just the right spot.

Also, there are two more stretches specific to this malady.

LEGS WIDE (IT BAND VARIATION)

1. Sit on the floor and open your legs to the sides. If you are not warmed up, let the straight knees relax and be careful how wide you go (remember the 80% Rule) (Photo 264).

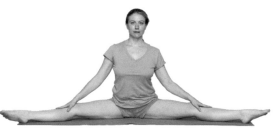

2. Supporting with the belly and the hands on the floor, take your body casually forward and around toward one leg (the working leg).

PHOTO 264

3. As you turn your chest to the working leg, lift your opposite hip off the floor as you roll your weight onto the outside of the working hip (Photo 265).
   Allow the opposite leg to relax and the knee to bend as necessary, following and turning in the same direction. You may rest the inside of your following knee comfortably on the floor, if you wish. (The entire role of the following leg is to accommodate without resistance.)

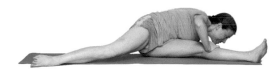

PHOTO 265   *PHOTO 266*

4. Supporting with your hands, chest facing the floor, bring your opposite shoulder to the floor, or as close as you can get, just beyond the working knee (Photo 266).
   If your weight is vertically aligned over the hip socket—and it should be by now—there is nothing more to say but, "voila!"

5. When you are ready, rise and approach the other side.

HEELS APART (HIP SOCKET) STRETCH

1. Sit on the floor and extend your legs casually. Leave them relaxed and flopped open.

2. Open your heels to, at least, hip-width apart (Photo 267).

3. Take your body forward and down, being sure to leave your legs passive (Photo 268).

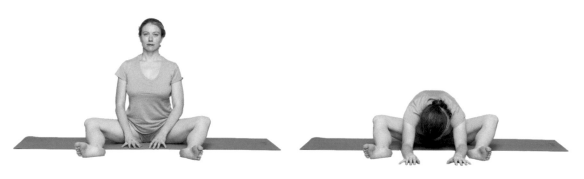

PHOTO 267   *PHOTO 268*

This will allow the knees and hips to bend and open, responsively, the farther you reach with your torso, putting the stretch itself into the hip sockets and the outside of the legs (the torso is the lever you move to work the machine; i.e., the hip sockets and I.T. band).

4. If you're hitting the right spot, hang out and breathe. If you're not quite there, adjust the width between the heels and, possibly, the degree of bend in the knees, until you're right on target.

5. Rise when you're ready.

Exercises:

For symptoms **1**, **2** and **3**, any and all exercises that feel helpful are fine. Symptoms **1**, **3** and **4**, should find reclining on the floor for **Crossover Crunches** (chapter VI) a fine place to start. Symptom **2** might do better beginning with **Squats** and **Lunges** (chapter VI).

After this, symptoms **1** and **2** can strengthen the area further with **Leg Lifts** (chapter VI). Symptom **4**, as mentioned in the Assessment section, is usually caused by weaker or less involved inner thighs. For this and **3**, proper **Lunges**, **Leg Lifts**, **Crossover Crunches**, **Open Cross-Cross** (chapter VI) and, if you can handle it, ballet plies will all help get your inner thighs on board.

THE LEGS, FEET AND TOES

THE THIGHS

As our legs are used primarily in a front-to-back motion, lifting from the top of the thighs and pushing from the back of the thighs, most of our injuries to these occur along these same lines. Some maladies of the thighs are actually symptoms related to causes in other areas and are best dealt with through **The Hips and Buttocks** and **The Lower Back** exercises. You need to look around.

SYMPTOMS

1. Increasing tightness, contracting knots, burning strains

2. Ropey pulling or a loose, disconnected feeling

3. Pain specific to one small area, or only in certain movements

ASSESSMENT

1&2.   These suggest muscles or tendons that were either overworked or not ready for a given challenge. You may cry out in agony the moment it happens, or not realize, until later, that something went wrong.

3.   This suggests one of two things:

A) A problem in structure and support, with the pain often felt at or near a point of connection between a muscle and its tendon, or in a tendon or ligament itself, especially where it attaches to the bones. This could be the result of overstress at a critical time, or grow slowly from regular, though even slight, misuse.

B) A telegraphed signal, from a nerve unhappy with its passage through a near or distant joint. (If this is the case, review the recovery techniques appropriate to the injury.)

WHAT TO DO

Massage:

1&2.   For large areas of sore muscles, something along the lines of Swedish massage, or deep-tissue massage, where the whole hands knead the whole mass like a hearty French batard, can offer great relief. However, if you're really tender, something comprehensive but much softer, like old-form Japanese Reiki, might make you a lot happier. For a happy median between these two, try a foam roller.

1, 2&3. For both large and small targets, acupressure (see **The Role of Acupressure**, from **Determining the Source of an Injury**, chapter IX) can be applied. If the injury is to the back of the thigh and you're seated, tennis balls can be brought into play.

(Before proceeding to **Stretches** and **Exercises**, see **Bandaging, Braces and Tape** section).

Stretches:

Back of the thighs: Similar to the hips and buttocks in their ability to both affect and be affected by the lower back, injuries to the backs of the thighs often involve one or both of these integrated neighbors. This allows the same stretching and strengthening techniques to be used, as they are all helpful, though the focus will shift more to those that are primary to the back of the legs.

The **Standing Hangover Stretch**, **Standing Bend and Stretch**, forward **Leg Swings**, **Knees to the Chest**, **Reclining Single-Leg Stretch** and **Cat Curl** (chapter VIII), and **Standing Single-Leg Stretch**, will be primary to your flexibility. A nice relief may be gained, as well, from the **Working Supine Stretch** (chapter II), depending on the nature of the injury.

If the **Standing Single-Leg Stretch** is too much, a gentler variation can be found in the **Seated Single-Leg Stretch**:

SEATED SINGLE-LEG STRETCH

1. Perform the **Seated Single-Hip Stretch**, both sides.

2. Return to the first side and extend the working leg along the bench (Photo 269).

If you are wearing shoes, let your heel hang off the end of the bench (the back of the shoe, when on the bench, elevates the heel higher than the bench seat and your hip, which can under-support, overstretch, and possibly strain, the back of the working knee and leg). Flex the working foot.

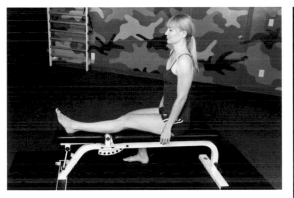 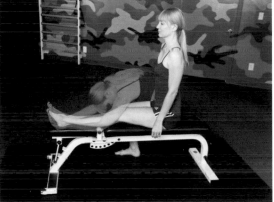

PHOTO 269

3. Reach out to the working leg with both arms—mind your neck and shoulders—drop forward and stretch (Photo 270).

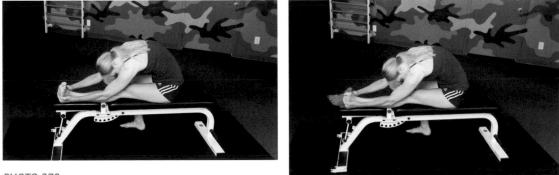

PHOTO 270

Point and flex a couple of times. Finish pointed (Photo 271).

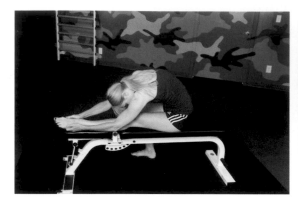

PHOTO 271

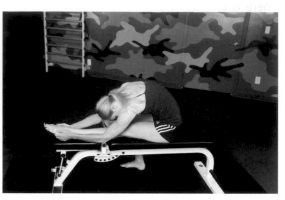

PHOTO 272

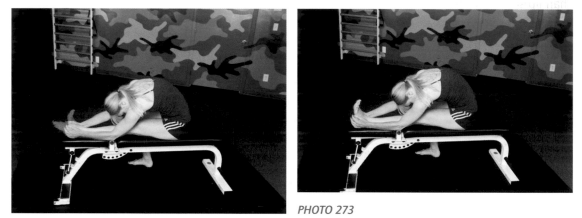

PHOTO 273

4.   Keep your upper body fully stretched as you rotate the working knee to the ceiling (Photo 272).

Flex and point a couple of times. Don't forget to work your toes.

5.   Roll the body up, exhaling and squeezing the belly, and change sides.

If you can't work this hard, or desire a more relaxing experience, both this stretch and its companion **Seated Single-Hip Stretch** can be done in almost complete passivity, excepting the belly should be engaged, mildly, at least, and the supporting leg should retain its alignment.

Front of the thighs: This is where we must change direction. Instead of hanging forward over straight legs, we now stretch or bend them behind us, with a torso that arches, and must be accounted for, as we do.

There is one standard stretch for the front of the thighs. I have seen it performed standing, lying supine on a bench, and lying on the side or with belly on the floor. I have rarely seen it employed to its full potential.

The idea is to bend the knee, grab the ankle and pull the leg backwards, therefore stretching the top of the thigh. Most people, however, just pull the working heel to the butt, which primarily stretches the lower end of the muscles, just above the knee, and not the muscles entirely. To stretch the muscles and their associated tendons thoroughly, bottom through top, one must try to pull the thigh behind the hips.

Problem is, an overtight top of the thigh is one of the most sensitive areas to stretch, and the combination of pain and the insecurity of a lower back forcibly arching, causes many to pay no more than lip service to the movement, which improves the situation little, if at all.

Standing, or lying supine on a bench, offer the best chance for both safety and muscular fulfillment in this stretch. Trying it lying on your side is unstable and might injure your lower back or hips. Trying it lying on your belly pulls the hips off the floor, again endangering your lower back.

Lying supine, on a bench, provides the most support. However, depending on the severity of your injury or the tightness of your quads, you may do better standing, where the stretch can begin at a softer angle, with less pressure. So, let's start there.

QUAD STRETCH (STANDING)

1. Face a supporting structure (a rail, bar, chair back, wall). Stand close enough to place the right hand on said support, without leaning forward, the elbow bent to no more than 90 degrees.

2. Bend the left (working) foot up to the back and take the ankle with the left hand.

3. Stretch the right (standing) leg, flatten your lower belly strongly, to protect your arching lower-back, and lift through the top of the head. Slowly and gently, pull the left foot up and back with the left hand (Photo 274).

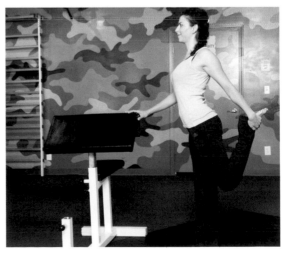

PHOTO 274

If you are tight, both draw the foot closer to the butt as well as drawing the left knee behind the line of the hips and the supporting leg. This stretches the entire top of the thigh, from its attachments at the hips and belly through its attachments to the top and sides of the knee.

If you are looser, and your foot easily bends to your butt, don't let it. Instead, engage the working thigh's muscles and press your foot into your lifting hand, as if to straighten your knee, distancing your heel from your butt as the knee moves behind the hips.

Extend your working elbow as you pull the working thigh back.

4.   Release and change sides.

Reclining on a bench may be a more challenging start, but the lower back is better supported and, if you can reach it, there is a point at which the stretch almost works itself.

QUAD STRETCH (SUPINE ON A BENCH)

1.   Lie supine on a bench. Bend your supporting knee (about 90 degrees), lift your foot and place it solidly on the bench, to protect the lower back. The supporting arm (same side as supporting leg) may extend along the bench and the hand may grip the bench for extra stability. The working foot is on the ground, the thigh roughly parallel with the floor (Photo 275)

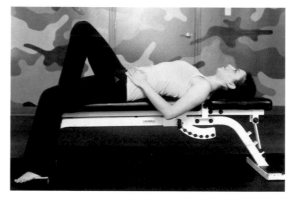

PHOTO 275

2.   Grab your working ankle with your working hand. Gently pull back, toward your butt, keeping the end of the working foot on the floor. Your working knee will continue to bend as it drops in line with, or below, the height of the bench (and, therefore, in line with, or behind, your hips).

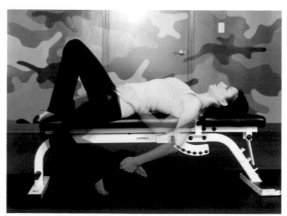

3. If tolerable, bend it back until the top of the working toes rest on the floor (Photo 276). As the floor's proximity to the height of the bench will now hold your working leg in this position, take the time to relax into the stretch and breathe.

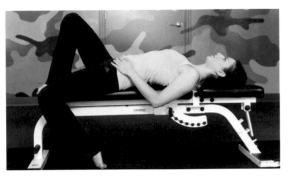

PHOTO 276

You will notice, at this point, that your knee and thigh are dropping below the height of the bench, and your back is beginning to arch. Support with your belly (squeeze) to take pressure off the arching lower spine.

4. Again pull the working foot back, if tolerable, until your stretch is complete (Photo 277). If it gives you something extra, you may pull your foot up against your butt.

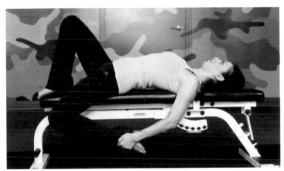

5. Carefully release the leg and go to the other side.

PHOTO 277

Exercises:

Crossover Crunches and **Leg Lifts** (chapter VI) should be beneficial to all symptoms, front or back of the thighs, with one consideration. In the case of an isolated point of pain, some movements will hit that wrong spot the wrong way, and these must be carefully avoided. Usually, a slight alteration of the movement—smaller or more supported ROM, knees rotated open instead of forward, flexed foot versus pointed—will relieve the stress and allow you to proceed.

From there, continue with **Squats** and **Lunges** (chapter VI). Remember the 80% Rule. For the top of the thigh, something along the lines of **Calf Extensions** (chapter VI) should be added.

THE KNEES

Injuries to the knee joint (tendon, ligament, cartilage, bone) result from misalignment (overstressed, under-supported), overuse or impact. Injuries to the small muscles at the back of the knee result from overstretch or an active strain. (Keep in mind, however, as with the thighs, sometimes pain in the knee is caused by injuries occurring elsewhere.)

SYMPTOMS

1. Pain just above the knee joint or along the sides of the kneecap

2. Pain behind the kneecap, or along its upper or lower edge

3. Pain behind, or shooting across the kneecap, especially when the knee is rolled side to side

4. Pain in the lower inside corner or lower outside corner of the joint

5. Pain above or below the inside or outside of the knee, or running the length from one to the other

6. Any of symptoms **1** and **2** from **The Thighs**, felt in the back of the knee

ASSESSMENT

1. This indicates a strain to the top of the thigh (the quads), most likely as it attaches to (wrapping down and around) the knee, involving both muscle and tendon.

2. This is usually brought on by one of four things:
    1. Extending the bent knee beyond the ends of the toes, as in an overaggressive forward lunge, or from habitually poor form climbing stairs or hills.
    2. Leaving the bent knee behind the heel when rising from a lunge or when climbing stairs or hills.
    3. Hyperextension of the joint, which also can engender symptom **6**.
    4. Plain, old impact, affecting the cartilage that cushions the ends of the bones.

3. This is a stability injury, usually from one sudden (though it may not be immediately felt), improperly aligned (rolling outside or in) misstep. It most likely involves the ACL, a ligament that crosses the knee to prevent wobble side to side.

4. This is a misalignment issue. At some point in one's movement, the bending knee is rolling— perhaps only slightly—either inside (lower inner corner injury) or outside (lower outside corner injury) of its alignment over the ball of the foot.

5. This is similar to symptom **3**. It tends to occur during rapid, impacting movements (track and field, uneven ground), when the ability to control the knee's alignment is less secure. Of course, if you're not paying attention, it could occur in a slower and softer situation.

6. This happy little number can show up just by overstretching the back of the knee, and you don't have to have hyperextended joints to cause it. If the muscles aren't ready for the stretch—pop

goes the weasel. Hard, straight-legged impact can also bring it on. An inability to fully stretch the leg, pain and weakness in certain movements is the result.

WHAT TO DO

Massage: As no large areas of muscle are involved, acupressure will serve you best. It will prove most helpful for symptom **1**, though some benefit may be found for symptoms **5** and **6** as well. symptoms **2**, **3** and **4** will benefit little from massage, unless the injury is found to include, or be instigated by, injury to the muscles of the lower back, hip, thigh or calf.

(Before proceeding to **Stretches** and **Exercises**, see **Bandaging, Braces and Tape** from **The Tools in the Workshop.**)

Stretches:

1-5.   Any stretches for the thighs, calves, feet and toes that help strengthen and align the knee. The **Working Supine Stretch** (chapter II), and the **Wall-Supported Hangover Stretch** reinforce stationary alignment, while the **Standing Bend and Stretch** (chapter VIII) challenge alignment and support through ROM.

6.   These can be accessed with any of the stretches for the back of the thigh, such as the **Wall Supported Hangover Stretch**, any **Single-Leg Stretch—Standing**, **Seated** or **Reclining**, the **Standing Bend and Stretch** and **Leg Swings** (chapter VIII).

Exercises:

1-6.   For stationary stability, **Standard Crunches**, the **Standing Calf Raise** and possibly **Leg Lifts** (chapter VIII). For rehabbing moving alignment, **Crossover Crunches**, **Calf Extensions**, **Squats** and **Lunges** (also chapter VIII) should give one plenty to consider.

Remember, pay close attention to form, especially at the transition from bending the knees to straightening them.

THE CALVES

Although the calves are subject to many of the same injuries as the thighs, they also claim a few particularly pernicious ones all their own.

SYMPTOMS

1. Any of the symptoms from **The Thighs,** either in the big muscles on the back of the calf, the Achilles tendon, or along the outside of the calf

2. An inability to flex the foot or sustain weight in the heel, with pain in the back of the calf when attempted

3. An inability to point the foot or rise up on the toes, with pain in the back of the calf when attempted

4. Pain in the back of the bottom of the heel, which burns upon impact or, in severe cases, merely by putting weight on it.

5. Pain, constant, throbbing, burning, or all three (lucky you), running along the vertical edges of the large bone in the front of the calf (the tibia), especially upon impact.

ASSESSMENT

1. Something wasn't ready, or strong enough, for the task at hand. If it's in the big calf muscles in the back, it's probably only muscular. If the pain is restricted to the Achilles, it may be just in the tendon, or caused by the calf muscles. (The Achilles can be a delicate piece of goods to rehabilitate.)
   If it occurs in the muscles on the outside of the calf, it's a stability issue, likely from uneven ground, moving side-to-side, multidirectional stress or uneven impact. One should check the knee, ankle and, possibly, foot for either causal (via the neural telegraph) or collateral damage.

2. This is an injury to the deeper muscle in the back of the calf, the one that—you guessed it—flexes the foot. It generally occurs from ballistic movement, the apparatus either being overstretched under duress, freezing up or just not stretching when called upon to do so, while supporting weight.
   (When it happened to me, it felt like a golf ball, at low speed, had hit the back of my calf. Not that big a deal. Ten minutes later, I could barely walk.)

3. This is an injury to the more superficial muscle in the back of the calf, the one that points the foot. It usually occurs from one rapid movement, or spending too much time on one's tiptoes.

4. Welcome to the world of Plantar Fasceitis, a very unhappy type of strain in the foot. In this case, though, the pain occurs where the Achilles tendon attaches to the bottom rear of the heel, the origins of the strain will most likely be found in the big muscles in the back of the calf. These,

over—or unevenly tightening, overwhelm the Achilles tendon and create a strain at its weakest point. In this situation, that point is its thin, spreading, fanlike attachment at the base of the heel. Repeated impact is a major player here (running is a common culprit), either overdone or poorly supported. In those more sedentary, it seems to occur through poor body mechanics in daily activities, such as walking, climbing stairs, and, perhaps, prolonged standing. Calves that are tight to begin with can be more easily affected.

5. "Shin Splints" is the name of the game, in which the connective tissue (the fascia) that secures the large calf muscle to the bone begins to weaken and tear. The muscle begins to loosen from the bone and wobble, more and more, with repeated or improperly supported impact. It is usually a result of running or jumping, without full involvement of the back of the leg and heel, in their role as shock absorbers, when cushioning and transferring the falling weight.

I first met Shin Splints when I began studying ballet. When I would come down from a jump, instead of working from my toes down into the floor through my heels (the right way), I tended to keep the weight in the front of my feet throughout. My heels would scarcely touch the floor, or bounce off it, when I landed. Both my heels, and the back of my legs, the grounding and power of my shock absorbing system, were being cut out of the equation. It took me six painful months, during which time I had to seriously restrict the height of my jumps, to get these muscles on board and become pain free.

If your pain is so severe that you find you cannot support yourself on your feet, you may have gone beyond shin splints and created stress fractures in the large bones of your calves. It doesn't seem to be common, but it can happen. Remember, never hesitate to see a doctor if you feel you should.

WHAT TO DO

Massage: Follow the guidelines for **Massage** from **The Thighs**.

For symptom 4—plantar fasciitis—start exploring with mildly pressured fingers (see **The Role of Acupressure**, from **Determining the Source of an Injury**, chapter IX). Begin at the back of a bent, relaxed knee, where the big calf muscles begin. Work your way down slowly, feeling for inconsistent texture within the muscles. When you find the lines of pain, take your time working down through the heel.

Once at the heel, try pressing, slowly, from above the back of the heel, down through the bottom of the Achilles, through its attachment and out toward the front of the foot.

Before proceeding to **Stretches**, **Exercises** and **Movement**, see **Bandaging, Braces and Tape**, from **The Tools in the Workshop.**

Stretches:

1-4.   Stretches that work for **The Lower Back**, **The Hips** and the **Back of the Thighs**, from **The Thighs**, work for the calves as well. Even some with a bent working knee, such as the **Seated Hangover Stretch** (**The Lower Back**), when the working ankle rests across the supporting knee, can affect pain in the calves. As injuries vary, so will the benefit of one stretch or another. You've got to shop around.

If your pain is in the back of the calf, go more with stretches for the **Back of the Thighs**. The greatest benefit will come when you flex your working foot, as the 80% Rule allows, either passively or actively, as you stretch.

If your injury lies along the outside of the calf, you might do better with open rotation at the hips and knees as you stretch. In addition to stretches referenced in the preceding paragraphs, both the **Heels Apart (Hip Socket) Stretch** with flexed feet, and the **Working Supine Stretch** (chapter II) may bring you surprising relief.

5.   As shin splints are not a muscular malady, and occur at the front of the calf, stretching will not do very much to allay the symptoms. Some relief may be gained, however, with hand-assisted, straight-leg, flexed foot stretches, such as the **Reclining Single-Leg Stretch** (chapter VIII) and the **Seated Single-Leg Stretch** and the flexing, pointing and ankle rotations of the **Toes, Feet, Ankles and Calves** (chapter II).

If you're dealing with really tight calves, an injured Achilles tendon or plantar fasceitis, you might want to be very ginger, indeed, about your first, exploratory stretch.

The safest way I know to test the stretch in your calves, and assess their ability to support weight, is the **Standing, Supported Calf Stretch**.

STANDING, SUPPORTED CALF STRETCH

1. Stand tall, before a (roughly) waist-high rail or bar. Stand close enough that you can hold it, hands shoulder-width apart, with your elbows at your side. Feet are together.

2. With the hands and shoulders taking some of the weight, slowly bend the supporting knee while sliding the working foot back along the floor. Keep the hips and body (weight) above the supporting heel and the working knee relatively straight.

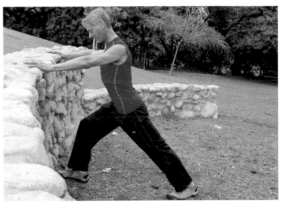

PHOTO 278

3. Keep the working foot's heel on the floor as it slides back (Photo 278). Stop when you hit the 80% mark, draw the foot back in as you stretch the standing leg and, whether it is suffering or healthy, work the other side. More than just to keep things even, you will find that the supporting calf gets a little—and different—stretch of its own.

If you cannot flex your foot, all of your early stage flexing stretches will have to be weight free and passive (hand, wall, or floor assisted).

MOVEMENT

1. Stay within a comfortable speed and ROM. Be careful of sudden drops and rises.

2. Stick with small steps, always leading with the injured leg, gently transferring the weight from one leg to the other (gain a cane if you must). Keep the knee of the injured leg relaxed and resist allowing your hips to get in front of the injured leg's heel, so as neither to force a flex in its foot nor put the bulk of the weight into the ball of its foot.
Lift strongly through the upper body to keep the load light. Stairs, or even a gentle rise in the terrain, require special attention.

3. Your walk will be similar to symptom **2**, though you may have a bit more freedom to move naturally.

4. Zero impact should be your goal. No running, no jumping, and only relaxed walking. Focus on full involvement of the foot, transferring the weight smoothly onto the forward heel as it reaches the ground, then securely through the length of the foot and on to the toes. Use your hips, knees and

ankles, in their supporting roles as the Lords Cushioner, the Absorbers of Shock, to come to the aid of their allies down south.

If you find, for some reason, that you must move rapidly, then move—I kid you not—like Groucho Marx. Very bent knees, smooth, low stride, no impact, no up and down bounce, always from the heels through the toes. (I managed to heal myself, through six months of this wretched affliction—all the while leading my boot camp, five days a week, in a one to three mile run, often over rough terrain—by running like Groucho Marx. I felt silly, I didn't have a cigar, but I managed to get a laugh out of some of my squad and I did recover from that nasty, nasty burning.)

5.   As with symptom **4**, no impact is the way to go. You may need to shorten your walking stride and slow it down a bit. Also, be careful about going up on your toes. You'll probably want extra support (hands on a bar or rail) when you first begin to rise onto these.

Exercises: For all symptoms, start off with less stressful forms, such as **Single-Leg Lifts** (chapter VI), until you see what you've got to work with (rotate your working knee open for best results). Keep the working foot flexed, for maximum stretch, or flex and point as your leg moves, for stronger exercise (pointing alone reduces the benefit to the calf in most cases). Then try **Open Cross-Cross** and **Leg Lifts** (chapter VI), again with predominantly flexed feet.

Heavier recovery comes with **Squats** and **Lunges** (chapter VI), and, for symptom **2** and, possibly, **3** (more gently), **Calf Raises**, either on the **Calf Raise Machine** or through the **Standing Calf Raise** (chapter VI).

Of course, walking, with full attention to detail, is essential to recovery from symptoms **4** and **5**, plantar fasceitis and shin splints. It's all about proper mechanics—practice minimizing impact, work firmly through your heels to your toes, transferring your weight smoothly from foot to foot, with pliant and supple shock absorption through your ankles, knees and hips, and, always, with excellent upper-body support.

THE ANKLE

SYMPTOMS

1. A sharp or nagging pain in certain positions or postures

2. Stiffness, tenderness, swelling, a diminished ability to support weight

ASSESSMENT

1. Something got too loose or too tight, usually from being left in one (mildly or strongly) stressed position for too long. Such injuries can come out of nowhere and be very annoying in the short term.

2. The ankle rolls, folks, that's its thing. A slight misstep, your weight's off center, your support gives way, you stumble and, often, fall. It usually rolls to the inside, dropping you out. But, depending on terrain, it could roll to the outside, dropping you in, with potentially harsher results, such as compromising the inside of your knee, your inner thighs and hips.

Severe injuries to the ankle—such as full tears, dislocations, compression fractures—often require medical attention. Nevertheless, though ankle injuries have different symptoms, once physical therapy is begun, recovery for an ankle tends to follow the same path.

WHAT TO DO

Massage: Start gently, well away from the epicenter, with soft, exploratory fingers (see **The Role of Acupressure**, from **Determining the Source of an Injury**, chapter IX). Work through the contributing muscles above the ankle (back, sides and front of the lower calf) and below (top and sides of the foot). Once you understand the problem, apply acupressure in these areas as needed.

Stay away from any swelling (see **Ice and Heat**, from **The Tools in the Workshop**). When it's down to mild inflammation, you can begin gentle massage in the area, if it feels helpful.

(Before proceeding to **Movement**, **Stretches**, and **Exercises**, see **Bandaging, Braces and Tape** from **The Tools in the Workshop**.)

Movement: You may not be doing a lot of this at first, leastways not on your feet. Remember, less can be more. It takes but one split second and one false move to shock your ankle and make things worse. So don't even get near such an opportunity.

Stretches and Exercise: These will go hand in glove. At first, there will be no weight on the ankle as you work.

ANKLE RECOVERY

PART ONE

1. Seated or supine, extend the working leg off the ground, either forward or vertical (see **Toes, Feet, Ankles and Calves**, chapter II). If you can fully straighten your working knee without hurting the ankle, do so for strength and control. This may prove easier with the knee rotated open.

2. Gently point and flex the toes. If this feels all right, softly add the ankles to the movement.

3. Do a few reps, maybe a dozen, as you explore your ROM (80% Rule).

4. When you're ready, you may attempt very small ankle rotations. Keep the pointing and flexing of your foot, during the circular rotations of the ankle, at a minimum, until you feel confident that increasing their intensity will do no harm.

5. Over the next few days, increase the strength involved in performing these three—pointing, flexing and rotating your ankle—while steadily increasing a secure ROM. As you work, place your strong, stable, working leg in different positions, such as changing angles of elevation, out to the side, and at different degrees of rotation from the hips. Different positions will subject the working ankle, and its muscles, to mild forms of the same stresses they will face when you're once again on your feet.

PART TWO

When it's time to try supporting your weight, if you can comfortably stand, walking will be your first challenge. If that goes well, you can move on to the **Standing Supported Calf Stretch** (see **The Calves**). From there, try the **Standing Calf Raise** (chapter VI). Take some of your body weight into your shoulders, through use of your hands on a rail or bar.

As the days pass, gently work your ankle back into your normal exercise routines. Take it slowly, never push it, have patience. The first day you feel great, like going for the gold, don't. Wait a little longer.

The best way to recover an ankle is through those activities for which it is used. Incorporating it into whole-body movements is essential for its return to normalcy.

THE FOOT

"All of those who can wiggle their toes, stand firmly un-defeeted."
—Anonymous

SYMPTOMS

1. Pain in one bony spot, on the bottom of the foot, when pressure is applied, whether moving or still

2. Symptom **1**, accompanied by a burning, or shredding sensation, especially when moving and in certain angles of stretch. This may also be accompanied by symptom **3**

3. Tightness or pulling along the bottom of the foot, usually along one particular line

4. A strain, tightness or sharp pain along the top of the foot

ASSESSMENT

1. You may have a bruised bone, but, more likely, you've strained something that crosses or attaches at that point.

2. Though usually occurring in the heel, plantar fasceitis can appear in other places on the bottom of the foot, but, once again, as with the base of the heel, it tends to show up at the connections of tendon and bone. Two prime locations are at the base of the big toe (the large pad under the front of the foot) and along the front of the arch, where it approaches the same location. In both of these, symptom **3** is a regular participant.
   An interesting aspect of this symptom is that it can manifest as collateral damage, from a pre-existing tightness in muscles along the back of the body, originating as far away as the lower back.

3. Something wasn't ready for the stretch, impact or movement and has pulled, knotted or strained. In such injuries to the bottom of the foot, it is easy to find the irregular tightness, knots (rare) and loosened ropes, of aberrant muscle fibers and tendon. There's not a lot of meat to contend with and the muscles tend to be long and thin.

4. This is a flexing injury, often accompanied by lifting the foot off the ground, caused either by prolonged stress or one shining moment. If it's near the ankle, there could be some rotational flexion damage as well. Farther out the foot, it's more likely to involve rising up on the toes and the flexing of the toes themselves.

WHAT TO DO

Massage: Acupressure, soft and exploratory to begin, then as the condition allows (see **The Role of Acupressure**, from **Determining the Source of an Injury**, chapter IX). For symptom **2**, review the method used for symptom **4** (plantar fasceitis in the heel), from **The Calves**. For the bottom of the foot in general, when seated, certain massage rollers or a tennis ball can help as well.

Though massage may not do a lot to help symptom **1**, if it's a bruised bone, some relief can be had, by working the area around the point of pain.

(Before proceeding, for symptom 4, and possibly for the arch of the foot, see **Bandaging, Braces and Tape** from **The Tools in the Workshop.**)

Movement: Look into cushioned shoe inserts. You can get them to support a weakened arch; with gel to soften impact in the heel and front of the foot; and cushioned overall. These give you an extra little margin of comfort and safety to more securely guarantee your recovery. As for the specific symptoms:

1. Lay off the impact.

2. Lay off the impact and rapid, or multidirectional, movement.

3. When climbing (stairs, hills), rely more on the hips and thigh. Keep the foot engaged but relaxed, only moderately flexed. When stepping upon it, bring it to the ground smoothly and transfer your weight into the grounded heel, before moving your weight forward and up, through the rest of the foot.

Stretches and Exercise:

1   Your regular routine will eventually work through the stiffness.

2-4.   See **Ankle Recovery**, from **The Ankle**.

THE TOES

SYMPTOMS AND ASSESSMENT

Toes get jammed into things, over-bent in both directions, sprained, strained, stomped on, mashed, separated and broken (see **Inflammation and Bruising**, chapter IX, and **Ice and Heat** from **The Tools in the Workshop**). In some cases, it is helpful to tape the injured toe to the one next to it, for added support and stability (see **Bandaging, Braces and Tape**, from **The Tools in the Workshop**). In severe cases, a splint is taped underneath the toe to inhibit movement.

WHAT TO DO

Massage: Even without swelling, inflammation or bruising, the injury may be too tender to manipulate directly. Unless you find one point where pressure seems helpful on the injured digit itself, you'll do better working the foot from the base of the toe down toward the heel. In severe cases, you may find relief of the pain and swelling from as far away as the calf at the back of the knee.

Movement: Walk with a shorter step, less bend and flex of the toes. Refrain from putting too much weight or pressure on the front of the foot. No sudden moves. If there is swelling or inflammation, wear a looser shoe or sandal, so as not to painfully squish anything and, whenever you can, elevate that foot above your waist.

Stretches and Exercise: Follow the same guidelines as for **The Feet** and **The Ankles**, just reverse the order of approach. Rather than starting from the toes to approach an injured foot or ankle (**Ankle Recovery**, Part One), start from the ankle, flexing, pointing, and rotating, to approach the injured toes.

THE ARMS, HANDS AND FINGERS

THE UPPER ARM (JUST HUMERUS)

SYMPTOMS

1. A tight gripping, burn or knotting in one spot, in the meat of the muscle or at either end

2. A loose or ropey feeling in the muscles

3. An isolated pain in the hollow of the elbow, or just above the back of the elbow

4. A single point, or line of pain, either along the inside or the outside of the bone of the upper arm, or just above, inside or outside the back of the elbow

ASSESSMENT

1. This can be caused by rapid-fire extension and contraction, repetitive stress, pressing or curling too much weight, one rep too many, that extra squeeze at full contraction, or, simply, one wrong move when you're dehydrated.

2. This is common, sometimes with a transitional burn, to rapid-fire extension and contraction, particularly with poor form and regular impact, as when working on a punching bag.

3. Both are muscular–tendinous maladies.
   In the hollow of the elbow, it usually involves a bundle or two of the muscle fibers in the biceps, straining the related tendons, resulting from an overtight moment that may or may not have occurred where the pain is felt.
   Just above the back of the elbow, look at the triceps and their tendons, though it could also signal symptom **4**.

4. The reward of one magic moment or, most often, repetitive stress. If the pain is isolated to one solitary spot, it could be a mild strain of the connective tissue (see plantar fasceitis, symptom 4 from **The Calves**, symptom 2 from **The Feet**, and Shin Splints, symptom 5 from **The Calves**).

More likely, however, for reasons yet to discover, is that you've got an unhappy nerve. Such injuries may be fairly localized, lying between the shoulder and the elbow-joints included, or involve everything from as far away as the lower back, through the neck or the base of the shoulder blade, out through the wrist and fingers. And, to make it more interesting, the actual site of the initial injury could lay anywhere along that path.

WHAT TO DO

Massage:

1&2.   In the meat of the muscles, use multifingered kneading. Out toward the ends and for the tendons, fewer fingers, smaller motions.

3&4.   This is an acupressure moment. Review it at **The Role of Acupressure**, from **Determining the Source of an Injury**, chapter IX).

Movement: As long as it doesn't hurt, you may move as you wish. Try to avoid sudden reactions and overstressed positions.

If your problem turns out to be repetitive stress, you might want to alter any deleterious habituations.

Stretches: If the problem is muscular, try the **Wall-**, **Self-** and **Couch-Assisted Passive Shoulder Stretch** (see **Shoulder Injuries**).

If the problem is nerve related, once you figure out the lines and extensions of your problem, review the applicable sections of **The Neck and Shoulders**, and the applicable sections of **The Elbow, The Forearm, The Wrist**.

For any of these injuries, the **Working Supine Stretch** and **Shoulder Rotation and ROM** (chapter II) may bring relief.

(Before proceeding to **Exercises**, see **Bandaging, Braces and Tape**, from **The Tools in the Workshop**.)

Exercises: The name of the game here is, "Don't overdo it." Unless you've really hurt yourself, most or all of your normal abilities will be available to you. Even if you must avoid certain positions for the moment, (many of) the exercises that hurt you can be the exercises that heal you as well.

1, 3&4. Lighten the weight, decrease your ROM, keep that form clean and limit yourself to a safe number of reps. (80% Rule)

2&4.   Slow it down. Smooth, controlled movement, shortened ROM, pure, clean form, a safe number of reps and lay off, or at least lighten, the impact for a while.

THE ELBOW

SYMPTOMS

1. Hard impact, whether directly smacked, or secondarily overcompressed, as when the locked elbow takes the impact, through the hand hitting the ground, to protect the body when one falls backwards

    Results may include, but are not limited to, soreness, stiffness, bruising, inflammation and swelling

2. Pain at the back of the elbow, specifically in the junction of the bones, particularly upon extension of the arm

3. Isolated, linear, or multiple points of pain above or below the junction of the bones, especially in certain movements

ASSESSMENT

1. You had an accident.

2. The joint has been overstressed, either by:

    1. hyperextension; or

    2. unsupported full extension: With resistance—poor muscular control at the arms' full extension, forcing the joints to either support the weight, as with locked elbows at the top of a **Push-up**, or hang freely, as from fully extended elbows at the top of a Lat Pull-Down. Without resistance—letting the uncontrolled throw of the joint stop the free-flying extension a punch, which literally jerks the joint apart.

3. These are symptomatic of injuries to muscles, tendons, and nerves, with maybe a little fasceitis garnish (see symptom **4** from **The Calves**).

WHAT TO DO

Massage:

1.   See **Massage**, from **The Ankle**

2&3.   It may not help as much for symptom **2**, but you won't know until you try. For both, see **The Role of Acupressure** from **Determining the Source of an Injury** (chapter IX).

(Before proceeding, see **Bandaging, Braces and Tape**, from **The Tools in the Workshop**.)

Movement and Stretches:

1&2.   Gentle extension and flexion, light work with resistance within a safe ROM (80% Rule) is probably all you can do to helpfully accelerate the healing process.

2&3.   See **Movement** and **Stretches** for **The Upper Arm**. These may only be of limited help for symptom **2**. If the pain extends down the lower arm, see the following appropriate section.

Exercises: See **Exercises**, from **The Upper Arm**.

THE FOREARM

Painful symptoms expressed in the forearms can be related to problems farther up (elbow or higher) or down the arm (in the wrists, hands and fingers). Though they may appear purely local, they often are not.

SYMPTOMS

1. A tight, knotted, ropey or burning feeling in the muscle or tendon, especially in certain movements

2. Specific points of pain, between the muscles and near their connections, or running down the forearm, possibly affecting the wrist, hand and individual fingers

ASSESSMENT

1. These injuries appear to be limited to the muscles and their associates, caused by resistance overload or repetitive stress, usually the result of a moment of weakness from above (the elbow), or below (the wrist).

2. These injuries can be combined with or symptomatic of poorly designed repetitive stress or over-loading at the wrist, elbow or shoulder or straining through the hands and fingers.

WHAT TO DO

Massage: See **Massage**, from **The Upper Arm**, and **The Role of Acupressure**, from **Determining the Source of an Injury** (chapter IX). Due to the relatively smaller size of the muscles of the forearm, their long, thin, linear design, and their roles in articulation of the wrist and fingers, fully understanding the extent of a problem here is of utmost importance to its complete and speedy recovery.

Here are a few helpful tips for acupressure:

1. Use the thumb of your opposite hand to work through the larger muscles on the inside of the forearm. Start in the hollow of the bent joint and work through all the muscles across the forearm, from one side to the other. In this fashion, work your way down the arm.

2. Use the fingers of the opposite hand to work the top of the forearm, in the same fashion, again starting from the elbow.

3. Using the fingertips and thumb, work down the inside edge of each forearm bone as well, top and bottom, from the elbow to the wrist.

(Before proceeding, see **Bandaging, Braces and Tape**, from **The Tools in the Workshop**.)

Stretches: The forearm stretches best from the wrist and fingers. See **Stretches**, from **The Wrist**.

Movement and Exercise: See **Movement** and **Exercise** from **The Upper Arm** and **Finger, Hand and Wrist Curls** (chapter VI).

THE WRIST

Unless your problem requires a surgical remedy, wrist injuries, however caused, tend to follow the same pathways to recovery. Exactly where the pain is, how it got there, and which stretches and exercises feel best, will vary.

SYMPTOMS

1. General soreness, likely stronger either on the back or the inside (palm side) of the wrist; often made worse by carrying weight, it can throb annoyingly all through the night

2. Sharp pain or numbness, especially at certain angles or when performing certain tasks (mousing around on the computer); frequently found in the company of symptom **1**.

ASSESSMENT

It depends on what you've been up to. These symptoms are causally interchangeable. Any, or all, can come from weight overload, overstretching, poor alignment, punching a bag, poor shock absorption (through the elbows and shoulders) when landing on the hands, carpal tunnel syndrome, repetitive stress—anything in which your wrist can be involved. Thought is required to trace the source.

WHAT TO DO

Massage: There is a technique that has special value at the wrist. Easy to perform, it involves nothing more than a brisk rubbing of the skin at the site of the injury. It seems to stimulate both the circulation of blood in the skin and the underlying, affected nerves, warming and soothing the area quite beneficially.

After this, acupressure (see **The Role of Acupressure** from **Determining the Source of an Injury**, chapter IX). Keep in mind that wrist injuries often form in collusion with trouble higher up. Do not fail to include **Massage** from **The Forearm**, which may lead your investigation even higher. Below the wrist, **The Hand** and, perhaps, **The Fingers** will warrant examination.

(Before proceeding, see **Inflammation and Bruising**, from chapter IX and **Bandaging, Braces and Tape**, from **The Tools in the Workshop**.)

Stretches:

STRETCH FOR THE BACK OF THE WRIST

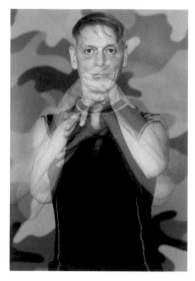

1. With your elbow at your side (not lifted out to the side), bring your left hand in front of the center of your chest, just above your solar plexus. Your wrist remains relaxed, your palm faces the floor.

2. Place the outside edge of your right hand, palm facing to the left, across the knuckles on the back of your left hand (Photo 279).

3. Lay your right palm down across the top of your left hand. Wrap the thumb and middle finger around the bend of your left wrist. The third and fourth fingers wrap softly into the palm. Leave your right index finger out of it altogether (Photo 280).

4. With a relaxed left arm and hand, squeeze your right thumb and middle finger together around the left wrist. Use them to lift your wrist vertically (no higher than the shoulders), simultaneously pressing down and to the left, across the back of the left hand, with the outside edge of the right hand (press toward the inside of the left forearm) (Photo 281).

5. Release to your starting position and do it again for 8 to 12 reps, both wrists.

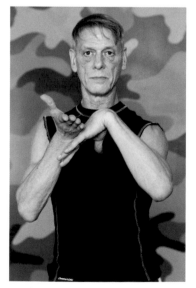
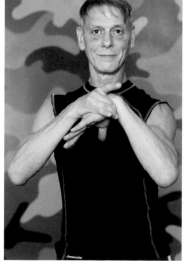
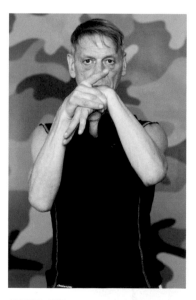

PHOTO 279   *PHOTO 280*   *PHOTO 281*

STRETCH FOR THE INSIDE OF THE WRIST

1. With your elbow at your side, lift your left hand. Place it in front of your chest, palm facing up, fingers forward (Photo 282).

2. Place your straight and strong right thumb into the center of the back of your left hand, just above the bend of the wrist.

3. Wrap the fingers of your right hand across the inside of the fingers of your left (Photo 283).

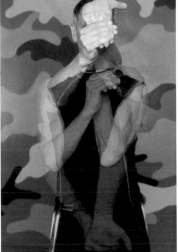
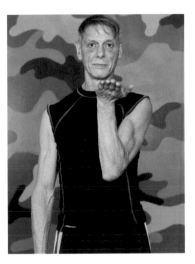

PHOTO 282

4. Pressing up and forward with your right thumb, pulling down and in with your right fingers (causing the left hand and fingers to arch), slowly extending the left elbow. For best results, try to take the left wrist, at its highest point, a bit above the height of the shoulders as you proceed (Photo 284).

5. Slowly take the hand out and down to the hips (Photo 285). Release and do your right wrist.

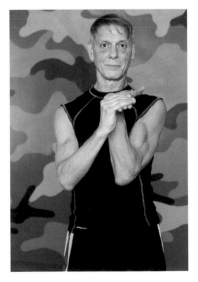
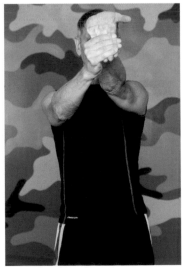
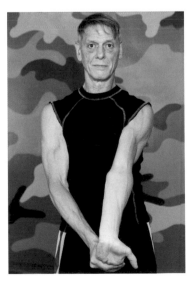

PHOTO 283   PHOTO 284   PHOTO 285

TWIST TO THE OUTER WRIST

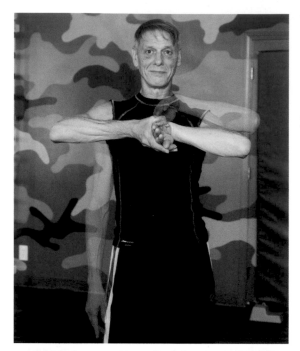

1. Lift your left elbow out to the side. Place your left hand in front of the center of your chest, just above your solar plexus, bend your wrist so that your fingers face forward (Photo 286).

2. Place your strong, straight right thumb over the middle of your left hand. Reach under your left hand with the fingers of your right, and wrap them into your left palm, around the base of the thumb (Photo 287).

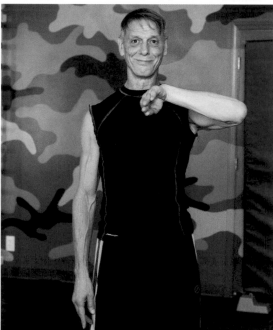

PHOTO 286

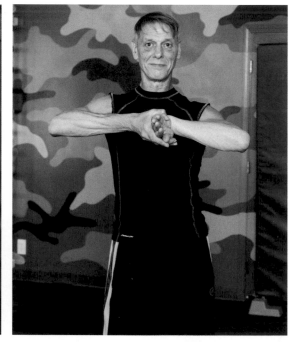

PHOTO 287

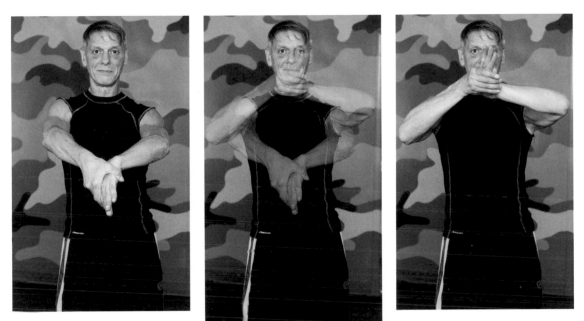

PHOTO 288   PHOTO 289

3. Reach forward and down, the right hand relaxing (Photo 288), before squeezing with the right, pulling up and back toward your chest, while twisting the top of the left hand to the right, with the thumb, while pushing the bottom to the left with the fingers (Photo 289).

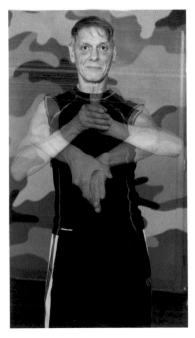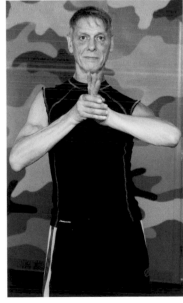

The stretch increases as the fingers are twisted vertically and the elbows bend (Photo 290).

4. Relax and repeat, eight to twelve reps, both left and right.

PHOTO 290

TWIST TO THE INNER WRIST

1. With your elbow at your side, bring your left palm up to your face, fingers vertical.

2. Place the strong and straight thumb of your right hand into the back of the left hand, just below the knuckles, between the third and fourth fingers (Photo 291).

3. Wrap the middle finger of your right hand around your inner left wrist, right in the bend. Wrap your third and fourth right fingers in to grip the inner left forearm. (Your right index finger remains aloof throughout.).

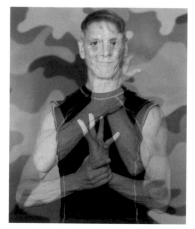

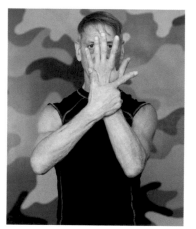

PHOTO 291

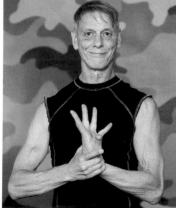

PHOTO 292

4. With the left arm and hand completely relaxed, press in with the right thumb, while pulling the left forearm down and twisting it open (away from the body) with the working right fingers. This will cause the left hand to corkscrew, or spiral, down and clockwise as it is pulled, stretching the wrist as it travels (Photo 292) (of course, were the right wrist being stretched, the right hand would spiral down counterclockwise).

5. Lift and repeat, for 8 to 12 reps, then do the right hand.

Movement: Be very careful about those things that cause pain. Recovery and reinjury share a razor's edge, especially in the hand.

Exercises: For isolating the muscles that work the wrist, see **Finger, Hand and Wrist Curls**, (chapter VI). Otherwise, your regular upper-body work should do fine, with one cautionary word—don't leave your wrists out of your work. They have a role to play, a strong holding position, a moving angle to match, a strengthened, safe alignment to achieve in every curl, punch, push-up, throw, swing, in whatever your arms are up to, and they don't get involved by themselves.

You must train your wrists, and your hands and fingers, too. This is the road to a safe recovery and a stronger, more dexterous, safer future.

THE HAND

SYMPTOMS
General soreness, sharp pain in one spot or with certain movements, a tight, knotted feeling (most often between the thumb and index finger), swelling, numbness, or any combination of these

ASSESSMENT
As with **The Wrist**, how your injury occurred depends on what you've been up to. Perhaps your hand got scrunched under the pillow for too long as you slept. Maybe it's from some kind of impact, or a strain caused by fingers that were lax, or unevenly stressed, under pressure. Perhaps the pain is secondary, a collateral gift from problems in the fingers, wrist or arm.

It's time for somber reflection.

WHAT TO DO
(Before Proceeding, see **Inflammation and Bruising**, chapter IX)

Massage: See **The Role of Acupressure**, from **Determining the Source of an Injury** (chapter IX). Now, here's a couple of handy (ahem!) tips when using it.

1. Start at the base of your inner palm with your opposite thumb. Work through the palm slowly, moving away from the wrist and toward the thumb and fingers. Start thus regardless of where your symptoms are. Remember, it's all connected, and this is progressively realized when working with something as intricately made as your hand.

2. A well-known way to relieve pain in the hand is by pressing into the meat of the muscle between the thumb and forefinger, squeezing from both sides with the thumb and fingers of the opposite hand. This works up to a point, but is easy to overdo, both by pressure and time spent squeezing. The same is true between the bones of the hand, especially just below the knuckles and above the knuckles, in the connections between the fingers. Sometimes less (80% Rule) is more.

Stretches: See **Stretches**, from **The Wrist** and **Finger Stretch**, from **The Fingers**.

Movement: As long as your fingers and wrist are all right, and you are willing and capable of properly using them, most or all of your normal ROM may be available to you. Don't push it, though, and don't overload the weight.

Exercises:

1. Gently squeeze the hand into a soft fist and release it again.

2. For exercise, using a soft and even resistance, such as a soft rubber ball or one of those bug-eyed stress reliever hand-squeezing novelties (no jokes, please).

3. Working the wrist, with or without weight (see **Fingers, Hand and Wrist Curls**, chapter VI). Also see **Tightening the Fist**, from **The Fingers**.

4. Anything your hand is capable of (80% Rule), properly supported, in your workouts or daily life.

Even with such age-related problems as osteoarthritis, employing these massage and exercise techniques regularly help keep your hands working at their flexible and dexterous best.

THE FINGERS

SYMPTOMS

Fingers get jammed, pulled and hyperextended at the joints (see **Inflammation and Bruising**, chapter IX), strained and, sometimes, knotted in the muscles. Their tendons can burn and tear (see **Bandaging, Braces and Tape**, from **The Tools in the Workshop**).

ASSESSMENT

These symptoms can occur singly or in combination. If your injury lies in a joint, you may remember when it occurred. If it's in the muscles or tendons, you might not have felt it happen. If the problem lies just with one or two fingers, it may have been caused by an uneven distribution of weight and support within the fingers, hand and, possibly, the wrist.

If the problem has been caused by habitual poor technique, that technique needs to be corrected.

WHAT TO DO

Massage: Even with no swelling or inflammation present, start with exploratory acupressure (see **The Role of Acupressure**, from **Determining the Source of an Injury**, chapter IX) in the palm of the hand. Work toward the knuckle and finger. Going into the finger itself may or may not be helpful. If it is, explore not only the top and bottom of the finger, but the sides as well.

Stretches: See **Stretch for the Inside of the Wrist**, from **The Wrist**, as well as the following.

FINGER STRETCH

1. Place your left hand, with a vertical palm facing to the right, in front of the middle of your abs. Extend your fingers vertically.

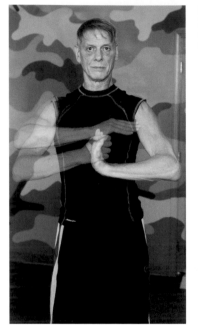
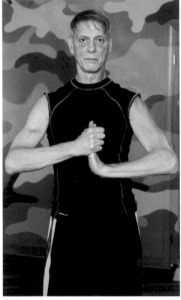
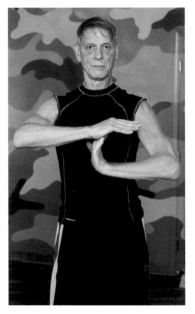

PHOTO 293   PHOTO 294

2. Place the palm of your right hand across the inside (palm side) of the left fingers and wrap your right-hand fingers around and across the back of the left (Photo 293).

3. Keep your left arm immobile by tightening the left shoulder. Using the right hand, press your left-hand fingers to the left, stretching back over (or, at least, toward) the back of the left hand and the left elbow (Photo 294).

4. Release and change sides.

Though your fingers can be stretched in this manner individually, be careful. It can be easily overdone.

Movement: This depends on your injury. If swollen and stiff—shorten your ROM. If strained or knotted, easy on the load.

Exercises: See **Exercises** for **The Hand**.

If your injury is from an improperly tightened fist and impact, do the following exercise.

TIGHTENING THE FIST

1. Stretch your palm and fingers vertically (Photo 295).

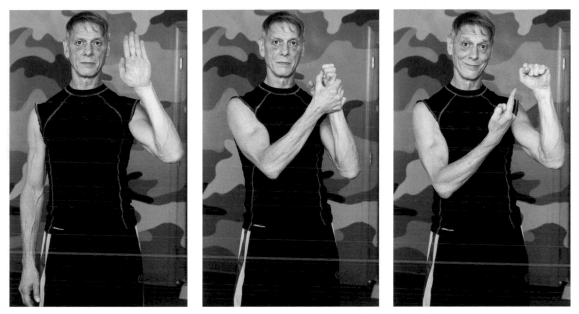

PHOTO 295   PHOTO 296   PHOTO 297

2. Keep the palm strong and straight. Bend you fingertips—one at a time, if possible—as tightly as you can, down into their bases. Try not to let the fingertips spill over into your palm. You may use your other hand to press the fingers into their bases more tightly (Photo 296).
    If you do, and you're new to this, expect a tight and stretched feeling over the backs of your bending fingers.

3. Once all four fingers are bent, roll your palm into a fist and squeeze strongly (the thumb remains outside, folding tightly across the backs of the middle of the fingers) (Photo 297).

IN SUMMATION

And so are presented the skills and techniques that have provided me, and so many of my clients and students, with a stronger and more healthful musculoskeletal system, an invaluable enhancement to so many aspects of our daily lives.

Whatever one may say about the joys and pitfalls of fate, I shall remain forever grateful to the many teachers of unsurpassed ability who have, so patiently and painstakingly, given such great benefit to my life.

Prominent among them are:

Osensei Hashimoto Shunjito, Sifu Jay Tavakollah, Sensei Robert Bryner, Fred Benjamin, Pepsi Bethel, Ms. Thelma Hill, Mme. Felia Dobrovska, Ms. Lynn Simonson, Mme. Darvash, Charles Moore and Mme. Albertine Maxwell.

My sincere thanks to them all!

Use this information they have given me. You'll be glad you did.

Keep in mind, though, that there is always more to learn.

CREDITS

Cover design: David Knox, Andreas Reuel

Photos: Derek Hutchison (derekhutch.com)

Layout: Andreas Reuel

Typesetting: www.satzstudio-hilger.de

Copyediting: Elizabeth Evans